PLASTIC

BODIES

EXPERIMENTAL FUTURES

Technological Lives, Scientific Arts, Anthropological Voices

A series edited by Michael M. J. Fischer and Joseph Dumit

DUKE UNIVERSITY PRESS

Durham and London

2016

Plastic Bodies

Sex Hormones and Menstrual Suppression in Brazil

Emilia Sanabria

Library of Congress Cataloging-in-Publication Data
Names: Sanabria, Emilia, [date] author.
Title: Plastic bodies : sex hormones and menstrual
suppression in Brazil / Emilia Sanabria.
Other titles: Experimental futures.
Description: Durham : Duke University Press, 2016. |
Series: Experimental futures: technological lives,
scientific arts, anthropological voices | Includes
bibliographical references and index.
Identifiers: LCCN 2015039926|
ISBN 9780822361428 (hardcover : alk. paper) |
ISBN 9780822361619 (pbk. : alk. paper) |
ISBN 9780822374190 (e-book)
Subjects: LCSH: Menstruation—Brazil—Salvador—Prevention. |
Hormones, Sex. | Contraceptive drugs—Health aspects—Brazil—
Salvador. | Menstruation—Social aspects—Brazil—Salvador. |
Menstrual regulation—Brazil—Salvador.
Classification: LCC QP263 .S263 2016 |
DDC 612.6/62098142—dc23
LC record available at http://lccn.loc.gov/2015039926

Cover art: David P. Wagner, Pill dispenser prototype for
oral contraceptives, 1962. Metal, plastic, wood, ¼ in. × 3⅛ in.
Gift of David P. Wagner. Image courtesy of National Museum of
American History, Kenneth E. Behring Center.

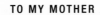
TO MY MOTHER

CONTENTS

ACKNOWLEDGMENTS

This book has been in the making for seven years. Its form has both endured and evolved through the encounters that continue to shape my thinking. Bringing it to completion has been a paradoxical process, one that—in a way—stands contra to its central thesis concerning the plasticity of things. Its present form is enmeshed in a lively web of conversations for which I am deeply grateful.

In Bahia, I was lucky to benefit from the support of the Gender and Health program (MUSA) at the Instituto de Saúde Coletiva (ISC) of the Federal University of Bahia. Thanks in particular to Cecilia McCallum, Estela Aquino, Greice Menezes, Ana Paula dos Reis, Jorge Iriart, Jenny Araújo, and Ulla Macêdo. Thanks also to João de Pina Cabral for transmitting his love of ethnography; to Luisa Elvira Belaunde, Elena Calvo-Gonzalez, Silvia De Zordo, Luis Nicolau Parés, and Ana Regina Reis for the inspiring conversations that helped shape this work; as well as to Rosário Gonçalves de Carvalho, Míriam Rabelo, Cecília Sardenberg, Graciela Natansohn, and Ileana Hodge. This work would not have been possible without the testimonies of the women who agreed to share their stories and insights with me, and I am deeply grateful for their generosity and openness. I am grateful for the patience and interest shown by the staff in the different medical and pharmaceutical sectors in which I was able to work, in particular, CEPARH and HEMOBA, and to Flávio Costa Pereira and Mauro Bitencourt, as well as to the members of the Association of Travestis of Salvador. Josefa Pereira da Silva deserves special thanks, as does Dona Nancí for her stories. Ivana Chastinet, Márcia Motta, Rose Rihan, Lise Silvany, Rose Silva, Rowney Scott, and the McCallum-Teixeiras taught me about much more than Bahia, and I thank them with all my heart for their friendship.

In the Department of Social Anthropology at the University of Cambridge I was lucky to benefit from the support of Marilyn Strathern, who is an exceptional teacher. I am deeply grateful for her patient guidance, care, and support. During my time in Cambridge I met wonderful scholars who would become dear friends, in particular, Charlotte Faircloth, Zeynep Gürtin, Ann Kelly, Ashley Lebner, Ayesha Nathoo, and Signe Nipper Nielsen. My heartfelt thanks to them for their friendship. I am grateful for the institutional and financial support provided by King's College Cambridge and the Economic and Social Research Council during my doctorate and the Fyssen Foundation and the École des hautes études en sciences sociales (EHESS) during my postdoctorate at the Institut interdisciplinaire d'Anthropologie du contemporain. At the École normale supérieure de Lyon, where I am now based, Frédéric Le Marcis and Samuel Lézé have been wonderful interlocutors. My thinking also owes much to the exchanges sustained with colleagues in the context of the Global Health: Anticipations, Infrastructures, Knowledge seminar at EHESS, Paris, as well as with colleagues of the editorial board of Sciences sociales et santé.

Anita Hardon read multiple chapters and followed with astute questions that helped me sharpen my arguments in key places. Working with her and the ChemicalYouth team at the Amsterdam Institute for Social Science Research has been a real pleasure and a marvelous opportunity to push my thinking about drugs and pharmaceutical efficacies further. I am particularly grateful to Kaushik Sunder Rajan for his encouragement, kindness, and friendship and for helping me see more clearly the underlying logic of the book. My heartfelt thanks to Emily Yates-Doerr for her friendship, care, and unfailingly smart advice, as well as to Alex Edmonds for his encouragement and for helping me clarify key ideas. I am grateful to the many people who read or listened and commented on versions of the chapters presented here and with whom I exchanged ideas in the course of this project: Nathalie Bajos, Julien Barrier, Claire Beaudevin, Barbara Bodenhorn, Charlotte Brives, Maurice Cassier, Simon Cohn, Michèle Cros, Philippe Descola, Stefan Ecks, Sylvie Fainzang, Claude Fischler, Soroya Fleischer, Daniel

Frandji, Sarah Franklin, Françoise Barbira-Freedman, Romain Garcier, Jean-Paul Gaudillière, Sahra Gibbon, Susan Golombok, Elena Gonzalez-Polledo, Françoise and Pierre Grenand, Miriam Grossi, Cori Hayden, Nick Hopwood, Julia Hornberger, Stephen Hugh-Jones, Frédéric Keck, Guillaume Lachenal, Patricia Lambert, Anna Lavis, Nicolas Lechopier, Sabina Leonelli, Ilana Lowy, Jonathan Mair, Daniela Manica, Daniel Miller, Annemarie Mol, Anne-Marie Moulin, Alex Nading, Haripriya Narasimhan, Yael Navaro-Yashin, Vinh-Kim Nguyen, Kristin Peterson, Maja Petrović-Šteger, Emmanuelle Picard, Laurent Pordié, Marie-Christine Pouchelle, Fabiola Rohden, Nick Shapiro, Susan Leigh Star, Eduardo Viveiros de Castro, and Umut Yildirim.

The insights, wisdom, teachings, and friendship of Bernadette Blin, Emilia Bucaretchi, Jan Day, Lily Defriend, Lucia Durante-Ringham, Josie Fenton, and Roberta Rodriquez have been an invaluable source of support and inspiration. I will never be able to thank my parents Laura Rival and Edgar Sanabria enough for enabling me to listen to and follow my heart. I am lucky to count Francine Sanabria, Martin King, and Pierrette and Daniel Chartier as what, in French, we refer to as *beautiful* parents, and I am deeply grateful to them, as well as to my three wonderful sisters, Chloé Sanabria, Lison Sanabria, and Léa Rival, for their loving care and support. Without Denis Chartier's love, wisdom, and boundless support I would not have been able to write this book. I am so grateful to be walking this path by his side. Birthing and nurturing our daughter, Luce Isadora, helped me deepen my understanding of bodily plasticity. The joy, light, and love she brings inspire me; I thank them both deeply for making the world so bright.

An earlier version of chapter 1 was published (in a different form) as "The Body Inside Out: Menstrual Management and Gynecological Practice in Brazil," *Social Analysis* 55, no. 1 (2011): 94–112. An earlier version of chapter 3 was published (in a different form) in French as "Hormones et reconfiguration des identités sexuelles au Brésil," in *Clio. Femme, Genre et Histoire*, no. 37 (2013): 85–104. A shorter version of chapter 4 was published (in a different form) as "From Sub- to Super-Citizenship: Sex Hormones and the Body Politic in Brazil," *Ethnos* 75, no. 4 (2010): 377–401. Small portions of an earlier version of chapter 5 were published in "'The Same Thing in a Different Box': Similarity and Difference in Pharmaceutical Sex Hormone Consumption and Marketing," *Medical Anthropology Quarterly* 28, no. 4 (2014): 537–55.

INTRODUCTION

PLASTIC BODIES

In June 1975 the *San Francisco Chronicle* and the *San Antonio Express* ran articles on a young Brazilian scientist's research on hormonal contraceptives. "I have declared a war on menstruation," Elsimar Coutinho, the Brazilian scientist, told the *Chronicle*, "his dark eyes flashing." The press coverage appeared in the wake of a meeting of the World Health Organization (WHO) task force on fertility regulation held in Texas. Coutinho told the *Chronicle*: "Before, we thought that lack of menstruation was a bad side effect of the long-term contraceptive pill. Now I consider it the main good effect (sic)." The *Express* reported that "he has patients in Brazil who have not had a menstrual cycle in 10 years." Coutinho is a polemical and highly mediatized doctor. Professor of human reproduction at the Federal University of Bahia's medical school in Salvador da Bahia (in northeastern Brazil), and director of a private research center and clinic called CEPARH (the Centre for Research and Assistance in Human Reproduction), Coutinho derived much prestige from the international networks he partook in throughout the 1970s and 1980s. Manica (2009) shows how he gained considerable local legitimacy through his international connections with institutions such as the Ford Foundation, Rockefeller Foundation, Population Council, and WHO, while opening up research hospitals (and their attending populations) in a strategic region for these institutions interested in the "population problem."

For years, he appeared weekly on women's television programs from where he professed advice about sexuality and family planning and found a unique platform to air his provocative statements such as, "Menstruation is a useless waste of blood" or "Eve did not menstruate."[1]

In 2005 I began fieldwork in Salvador with the intent of studying the role that sex hormones play in contemporary social life. I gained access to CEPARH, where a wide array of different hormonal regimens and treatments continue to be administered to prevent unwanted pregnancies, suppress menstruation, regulate moods, maintain youth, or assist reproduction. CEPARH is an atypical institution in the Bahian medical landscape, catering simultaneously—although in clearly differentiated spaces—to a clientele with private health insurance while offering a free, charitable family planning service to the "poor." On one of my first days at CEPARH, Dr. Paulo, one of the clinic's directors, took me on a tour. We began downstairs in the *ambulatório* (outpatient clinic), where a bustling crowd of women was waiting. "They come here from the *periferia* [slums]," Dr. Paulo tells me. "We give them high-quality *atendimento* [care], entirely for free." In the infirmary we met the two nurses who weigh patients, apply the contraceptive injections, and "release" the drugs that the doctors have prescribed. An old-fashioned glass cabinet full of jumbled pill and hormonal injection boxes occupies one wall, next to an imposing manually counterbalanced weighing scale. Faded advertisements for different hormonal contraceptives representing tenderly embracing, white, fair-haired couples hang on the wall. A framed photograph of a cesarean delivery sits on the desk next to a little figurine of a nurse holding a bottle labeled *carinho em gotas* (care in drops). One of the nurses is drawing the air out of a syringe while joking with a young, high-heel-clad doctor. Dr. Paulo introduces me and they nod knowingly. We engage in small talk: Larissa, the nurse, tells us that menstruation is *uma coisa muito moderna* (a very modern thing). Her grandmother only menstruated three times, she explains, her first period came when she was eighteen, then she had seven children, and by the time she was done, she was *menopausada* (in menopause). "Just like *as indias* [indigenous women]," Dra Beatriz added, "they never menstruate either."

Upstairs, CEPARH functions as a state-of-the-art gynecological center, where women who subscribe to private health insurance are offered a host of diagnostic exams and gynecological surgeries, and where doctors prescribe the newest contraceptive technologies, including tailor-made hormonal implants. The paint is fresher; there is air-conditioning and no crowds. A few days earlier, I met with Elsimar Coutinho in his office on the third floor. It is spacious, and I count nine statues of naked women, some neoclassical in varying shades of gold, several celebrating the pregnant form. I was invited to sit on a predictably low-lying sofa at the other side of his desk, behind a barricade of papers and journals. An enormous three-dimensional model of the female reproductive organs and a few glossy pharmaceutical monographs on new hormonal regimens sit on the coffee table beside me. After reviewing my research proposal, Coutinho noted that they needed more research on the "social" side of things. *Crendices* (beliefs) about menstruation still inhibited the uptake of the new hormonal contraceptive methods they have been developing at CEPARH. "You see, women don't understand yet that they have a *fake* menstruation when they use the pill. Pill makers used to instruct women to take a pause every 21 days to produce an artificial withdraw bleeding episode that women think is menstruation. But it is not menstruation, it is not natural and not necessary," he told me in impeccable English.

Menstrual suppression, or the idea that regular menstrual cycling is a new and potentially harmful phenomenon, received much attention globally after the 2003 U.S. Food and Drug Administration (FDA) approval of Seasonale, a contraceptive pill repackaged to produce only four menstrual periods a year ("Seasonale®. Fewer Periods. More Possibilities."), and the publication of the English translation of Coutinho's controversial book, *Is Menstruation Obsolete?* (1999).[2] Widely discussed in medical publications (Association of Reproductive Health Professionals [ARHP] 2004a, 2004b, 2006; den Tonkelaar and Oddens 1999; Edelman et al. 2007; Estanislau do Amaral et al. 2005; Ferreroa et al. 2006; Makuch and Bahamondes 2013; Thomas and Ellerston 2000) and global popular media (in particular, Gladwell 2000), the menstrual suppression debate is founded on two interconnected claims.[3] The first consists in differentiating the menstrual bleeding pattern experienced by oral contraceptive pill users from "natural" menstruation and suggests that the former, because of its artificial nature, is dispensable. The second claim denaturalizes regular menstruation, arguing that this is a "new biological state" (ARHP 2004b), since "in the past" or in "tribal" contexts women reached menarche later, had more children, and breastfed them longer than "modern" women do. Indirect evidence, this literature argues, suggests that this increases the likelihood of gynecological cancers and menstrual symptoms—problems purportedly overcome by the uninterrupted use of hormonal contraceptives.

Effectively, Seasonale—like the extended-regime pills used in Brazil—is nothing more than the standard oral contraceptive pill, repackaged. Since its inception in the early 1960s, the pill—as a set of daily tablets—has been "unpacked," and is better conceived in terms of the synthetic hormones that compose it. It has given way to a multitude of products in different forms of packaging and with different modes of administration. First, there is a profusion of orally administered pills—combination (estrogen and progesterone), mini-pills, extended-regime, or "morning after" pills—associating any variation of the plethora of synthetically produced hormones. These can in turn be brand-name drugs produced by international pharmaceutical laboratories, or copies of these (Sanabria 2014). In addition to this profusion of oral forms, contraceptive sex hormones may be injected (in monthly or trimonthly doses, such as Depo-Provera); implanted subdermally (such as Implanon); or absorbed through the skin (via transdermal patches such as Ortho Evra, creams, or gels), the vagina (via the vaginal "ring" Nuvaring), or the uterus (via the intrauterine hormone-releasing "system" Mirena).[4] These changes in modes of administration produce different drug entities, but also different kinds of consumers, bodily effects, and subjectivities. Many long-acting hormonal methods intercede in the "normal" monthly bleeding episodes experienced by women. This requires that women be "educated" or "counseled," to borrow the terms used by the ARHP (2004), to recognize the positive benefits of menstrual suppression, a task that Coutinho has carried out with astonishing determination throughout his career. In this book I examine the ways in which "the" pill has been unpacked and turn my attention to what is done with hormones as they are put to new uses, reassembled and then released from their packages and ingested or otherwise absorbed into bodies.

Four in five American women (82 percent) have used the pill at some point (Daniels et al. 2013) and 23 percent have used the hormonal contraceptive injection Depo-Provera.[5] In Brazil, 49 percent of sexually active adolescents use the pill (Rozenberg et al. 2013), as do 27 percent of women in a relationship. This makes the pill the most used method, just ahead of female sterilization. Today over 100 million women worldwide use hormonal contraceptives, and 80 percent of women of reproductive ages in Western Europe and the United States are considered "ever-users," making the pill one of the most widely prescribed drugs in the history of pharmaceuticals (Brynhildsen 2014; Tone 2001). Sex hormones have become key therapeutic agents in women's health and are central to contemporary understandings of the body, sex, and personhood. Yet, despite their ubiquity, sex hormones have seldom been studied ethnographically. Existing work on sex hormones tends either to be historical (Gaudillière 2004; Marks 2001; Oudshoorn 1994; Soto Laveaga 2009), to focus solely on North American contexts (Jones 2011; Kissling 2013; Watkins 2012), or to focus on how knowledge is constructed around sex hormones (Dos Reis 2002; Fausto-Sterling 2000; Löwy and Weisz 2005).

Plastic Bodies provides an ethnographic account of sex hormone use in Bahia, examining how hormones are enrolled to create, mold, or discipline social relations and subjectivities. Hormones are hybrid, complex objects that cut across political and sexual economies and sit at the boundary between sex and gender. This book considers the way the scientific concept of "sex hormones" is materialized into pharmaceuticals and how, as drugs, hormones leave the laboratory and are taken up by users and absorbed into everyday understandings of the body. As an anthropologist, I am interested in making visible the social relationships through which sex hormone uses are legitimized and in showing how these relations in turn mediate the lived effects of hormones. Plastic Bodies thus attends to the materiality of sex hormones while arguing that their efficacies cannot be reduced to their pharmacological properties.

The book tells two intertwined stories: the story of hormonal menstrual suppression and a story about bodily plasticity and malleability. Drawing on in-depth interviews with women, doctors, pharmacists, and health planners, I show that the locally prevalent practice of menstrual suppression grew out of Cold War neo-Malthusian concerns with overpopulation in the Global South. In recent years it has been remarked into a practice of pharmaceutical self-enhancement couched in neoliberal notions of choice and control. I map the specificity of these coexisting biopolitical rationalities in Bahia through an analysis of the peculiar local context of experimentality (Petryna 2009), aspirational class dynamics, and showbiz culture (Edmonds 2010), and by reference to the role that consuming medical services and being knowledgeable about health play in constructing social relations. The book adopts an object-centered approach that enables me to study both private practice medicine and public health institutions and to examine the different ways hormones are prescribed and adopted by upper-middle-class or low-income women. These conversations are often kept apart in anthropologies of Brazil (e.g., Biehl 2005; Scheper-Hughes 1992). Plastic Bodies is concerned with the way biomedicine and modernity are embroiled in Brazil (Browner and Sargent 2011; Caldeira 2000; Clarke et al. 2010). Inspired by the pharmaceutical anthropology literature (Whyte, van der Geest, and Hardon 1996, 2002), I followed hormones around, in women's descriptions of menstruation and of the body, in ideas about blood, and in a variety of medical and pharmaceutical contexts. I set out to examine what happens when this biomedical concept travels, reconfiguring lay understandings of menstruation, reproduction, and the body. My questions about hormô-nio—as it is referred to locally—were met with statements about sexuality, gender relations, and reproduction, and elicited discussions concerning hygiene, bodily interventions, and modernity. The ethnography opened into a range of related questions concerning the role of medical institutions and regimes in the making of citizenship. Adopting an object-centered or "follow-the-thing" approach (Appadurai 1986; Haraway 1991; Marcus 1995; Martin 1994), I traced the circulation of pharmaceutical sex hormones, as manifestly material objects, and their associated discourses through a range of contexts. This study of sex hormones as "things medical" (Clarke et al. 2010, 380) or materia medica (Whyte, van der Geest, and Hardon 2002)—read through the stratified Brazilian biomedical system—sheds light on how hormones are mobilized within contemporary biomedical regimes (Foucault 1976). As contraceptives, sex hormones are central to demographic interventions at the level of the population, and through the unfurling of new forms of administration, sex hormones are entangled in the individualizing modes of biopolitics, concerned with the disciplining of subjectivities and the performance of the body at the molecular level.

Drawing on an analysis of local understandings of blood and menstruation, and of the role of medical institutions in Brazilian social life, Plastic Bodies examines why the body is so readily made open to biomedical intervention in Brazil. The book argues that this can be explained by the fact that the body is understood to be malleable and plastic. It shows that, rather than breaching the body's boundaries, medical interventions are integral to producing the body and its delimitations. In his ethnography of plastic surgery in Rio de Janeiro, Edmonds (2010, 66) argues that Brazilian modernity is an aspirational process, perceived as always incomplete: "The modern is not quite now, but rather a goal that is continuously receding." This gives medical techniques a particular "mystique" that Edmonds (2010, 67–68) qualifies as a fetishism of technological progress, often driven by mediatized doctors. Malcolm Montgomery, who is famous for his cover stories in Brazil's Playboy magazine and regular appearances in people magazines, where he is presented as the gynecologist of the "stars," is a fervent defender of hormonal treatments. In an interview I carried out with him, he relayed to me his tale of two sisters: the *natureba* (a derogatory term for "naturalist") and the *high tech* (in English, in our conversation). The first, who is a hippy, went to live on a farm and had four home-births and breastfed for years. The second is a "beautiful businesswoman," had two elective cesarean births followed by plastic surgery, and did not breastfeed. The latter is his patient and, at her fortieth birthday, he recently met her sister, younger by one year but "looking sixty, at least," with her graying hair, collapsed breasts, and—he posited—prolapsed uterus and *rasgada* (torn) vagina. Natural births, he told me, are violent and aggressive; they distend the vagina and damage the perineum. They are "*um espetáculo de miséria estética* [a spectacle of esthetic misery]," he concluded. He narrated to me his experience traveling to the United States for a medical conference in the 1980s, during which feminists had marched "against the pill." Why would women march against themselves, against their own autonomy, he had wondered?

This intrigued me. Such people have a very naïve view of nature. Nature is aggressive. We had to fight against nature to achieve our quality of life, to have a better life. That thing that Rousseau said about living in harmony with nature, I really don't agree. . . . It is an error to think that, naturally, women should menstruate. It is biologically correct for women to have roughly between forty and eighty cycles in her life. A modern woman like you will have an average of two children and menstruate uselessly around 400 times. And this is why it is medically interesting to use *anticoncepcionais* [hormonal contraceptives] to lower the doses of hormones that naturally occur when women cycle. The doses administered in anticoncepcionais are immensely inferior to the natural peaks that occur when women cycle and which lead to a host of pathologies. Technology is important to adapt to the hostile natural world.

As I explore in this book, the appeal to the distinction between nature and artifice carries, in Brazil, particular values concerning the modernization of the nation, a project intimately tied up with questions of reproduction (Edmonds 2010). Writing from North American or Western European contexts, some authors have argued that recent developments in the biotechnologies reconfigure or "denaturalize" the idea of biology in its relation to the social. This book shows how, in Brazil, this is not new (Rohden 2003, 2001), as nature is already understood to be plastic. Mapping the class and gendered distribution of the prescribed and improvised hormonal regimes adopted by people in Bahia, it opens up a series of questions concerning the relation between self-improvement, control, hygiene, biomedical citizenship, and the Brazilian project of modernity.

Unmaking "the" Pill: Sex Hormones and Menstrual Suppression

Historical analyses of steroid sex hormones' disparate configurations in biomedical practices past and present reveal that these are particularly fluid objects (de Laet and Mol 2000). In the mid-1920s sex hormones were involved in clinical trials for menstrual irregularities. In the initial marketing strategy, the contraceptive qualities of hormones were presented as a side effect. The development of these therapies into "the" pill came late given the range of medical indications for which they were being used. One could argue that this played a significant role in the establishment of flexible therapeutic indications for these newly developing pharmaceuticals. This demonstrates the complexity involved in dealing with such objects. The pill, hormonal therapies, or fertility treatments are not natural kinds or categories that we can refer to without evoking their context. Sex hormones, in their form as pharmaceuticals, are made into particular kinds of objects by the social relations within which they exist.

"The" pill was initially dispensed in a glass bottle containing fifty tablets, and issued with directions on how many tablets to take and how long a pill-free interval to count in order to reproduce a monthly cycle. Couples are reported to have placed the pills on calendars to facilitate counting, and in the early Puerto Rican trials "illiterate" women were issued rosaries as counting aids (Gossel 1999). The circular Ortho-Novum dispenser released in 1963 was based on the patent delivered to David Wagner for his pill administration mechanism. This served to stabilize, within the pill's design, a regular menstrual cycle of twenty-eight days. It is interesting that what Akrich (1996) terms the "temporal coordination apparatus" was built into the pill's design *after* the drug was launched as a contraceptive and is not intrinsic to its design. The consolidation of this artificial bleeding episode was further stabilized through a series of changes that were made to the pill's dispensing mechanism. Thus, the pill came to include dummy or placebo pills, often containing vitamins or minerals, during which women experienced a "mock" — or fake — period. Historically, the monthly withdraw bleeding period experienced in the pill-free (or placebo) interval was considered im-

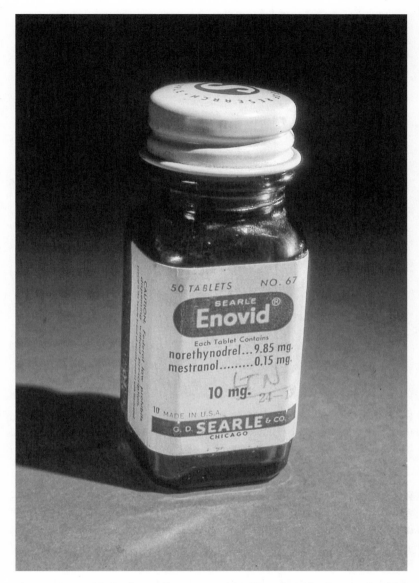

Figure I.1 Enovid, the first oral contraceptive pill approved by the FDA in 1960, was dispensed in a bottle of fifty tablets. Image credit: Smithsonian Institution, National Museum of American History.

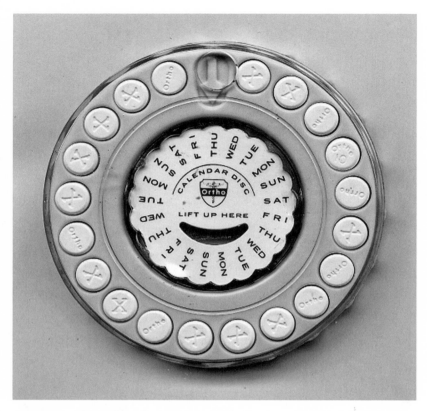

Figures I.2 and I.3 The Ortho-Novum 21 DialPak (1963), and its patent, introduced the notion of a cycle into the pill's design. Image credit: Smithsonian Institution, National Museum of American History.

portant for a variety of reasons, by both users (for whom regular bleeding was a sign of nonpregnancy) and doctors who promoted the pill as a form of "natural" contraception in its early days (see Gladwell 2000). It is just another step within this logic to move from scheduled monthly to seasonal bleeding intervals. As we have seen, the extended-regime pill Seasonale provides pills for a "3-month cycle": eighty-four pink active pills and seven white inactive pills. Interestingly, in Brazil only a minority of oral contraceptives include placebo pills, and women are routinely instructed that they can either take a seven-day break or *emendar cartelas*, which means beginning the new pill pack immediately without taking a break. This is facilitated by the fact that women can readily obtain pills over the counter in pharmacies

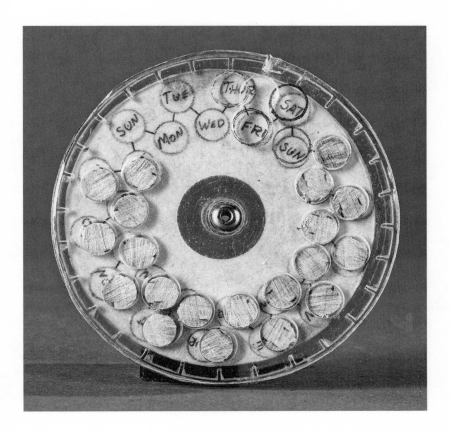

without a prescription, giving them greater flexibility in how they use the drugs. This explains why Brazilian women have long been experimenting with extended regimens to skip a period at their convenience, for a party, carnival, or a beach holiday.

The global circulation of sex hormones contributed to deconstructing the pill as a unitary object, either through the development of new forms of administration or packaging design, or through the widening of its field of action to include new indications, such as hormone replacement therapy, skin treatments, and "emergency" contraception. Oudshoorn's (1994, 1996, 1997) historical work on hormonal contraception provides a context to understand the dynamic of repackaging that I am foregrounding here. She argues that the history of sex hormones is a history of "Western science ignoring the local needs to specific users" (Oudshoorn 1994, 150–51) and traces the demise of the "one size fits all" approach to contraception

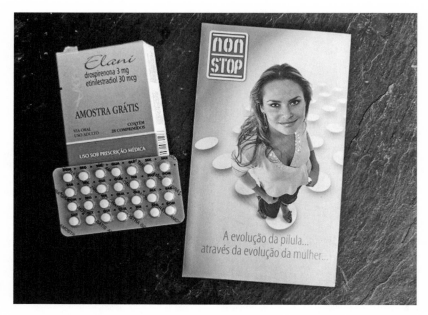

Figure I.4 Elaní is a widely available, fourth-generation extended-regime pill produced by the Brazilian pharmaceutical laboratory Libbs. "Non-Stop, The evolution of the pill through the evolution of woman" is a short information guide produced by Libbs to relay the idea of the evolution of the pill's design alongside women's evolution in society. Photograph by Emilia Sanabria.

promoted by early developers of the pill (Oudshoorn 1996). This led to the development of a "cafeteria model" of hormonal contraceptive diversity.[6] In the late 1970s the WHO actively promoted research on long-acting hormonal contraceptives such as hormonal injections and implants. These were seen as efficacious tools for population control programs because they are provider-administered. This makes them good "technical delegates," that is, artifacts that are "designed to compensate for the perceived deficiencies of [their] users," such as women's tendencies to forget to take their pills daily (Oudshoorn 1997, 44). The WHO research and development program stemmed from the recognition that "the pill" had only been taken up by "middle- and upper-class women in the western industrialized world." Injectable contraceptives such as Depo-Provera are described by the WHO team in a *Science* publication as particularly "appropriate in developing countries" (Crabbé et al. 1980). This logic was particularly evident in the Bahian public *ambulatórios* where I carried out my research, as I detail in chapter 3. The problem with long-acting hormonal methods is that they interfere with women's menstrual cycles, which explains, I argue, how the story of hormonal contraceptive development became entangled with the story of menstrual suppression. Gradually, the menstrual-suppressive side effects of the new modes of administration developed for the Global South were rescripted as desirable, primary effects. "Menstruate: What For?" was the title of a recent pharmaceutical industry-funded electronic newsletter (SaberMulher) that pinged into my inbox, explaining the health benefits of using long-acting hormonal methods to mitigate premenstrual symptoms. As discussed in detail in chapters 2 and 5, the lifestyle and esthetic effects of hormonal contraceptives gained much coverage in Brazil in recent years.

Contraceptive technologies, like any technology, are inscribed during their development such that representations of future users are materialized into the design of new products (Akrich 1996; Hardon 2006). They contain a configured user (Oudshoorn 1996) that can inhibit their capacity to travel. For the object to travel, a certain amount of context must travel too, so to speak. Failing this, the object is transformed as it is re-localized. For the pill to travel, it needed to be unpacked. As new objects were produced from sex hormones, their circulation worked to differentiate between different consumer populations. This background is important for understanding how choices are presented in reproductive health centers and clinics in Salvador.

DeGrandpre (2006) argues that the efficacies of drugs are informed as much by the cultural scripts that shape user expectations as by the drugs' pharmaceutical properties. As a pharmacologist he is uniquely placed to advocate that his discipline is "not equipped to grapple with the powerful dialectic that exist[s] between drugs, their users, and the historical and immediate contexts of use" (237). He argues that lay and expert understandings are infused with a kind of magicalism that assumes that the effects of drugs reside entirely in the substance, reducing understandings of pharmaceutical efficacy. Plastic Bodies examines the unwritten cultural scripts or "placebo texts," as DeGrandpre refers to them, that accompany and shape sex hormones use in Brazil. It does so while simultaneously taking seriously the material efficacies of hormones, attending in ethnographic detail to how hormones "retool sensuousness" (Hayward 2010, 227) by immersing "the body's organs in a chemical bath such that one's proprioceptive sense is . . . changed" (229). The lived experiences of hormones related by people I encountered were widely shared, attesting to a particularly powerful convergence between such proprioceptive retoolings and their attendant cultural

Table 1.1 Menstrual Suppression Methods Available in Salvador

Type of method	Brand name	Active principles
Extended-regime oral contraceptive pills	Elaní (Libbs Brasil)	Drospirenone 3 mg and ethinylestradiol 30 mcg
	Gestinol 28 (Libbs Brasil)	Gestoden 75 mcg and ethinylestradiol 30 mcg
	Any monophasic, combined oral contraceptive pill taken without the 7-day pill-free interval. Options range from Microvlar (Schering) and its "similar" Ciclo 21 (União Quimica) (0.03 mg ethinylestradiol and 0.15 mg levonorgestrel) to Yasmin (0.03 mg ethinylestradiol and 3 mg drospirenone).	
Trimonthly injections	Depo-Provera (Pfizer) or Contracep (Sigma Pharmaceuticals), Depo-Provera's Brazilian "similar"	Medroxyprogesterone acetate: injectible suspension of 150 mg/mL
Subdermal hormonal implants	CEPARH's "tailor-made" implants	Presented in capsules of testosterone, estradiol, gestrinone, elcometrine, levonorgestrel combined according to required dose.
	Implanon (Organon)	Single subdermal implant containing 68 mg etonogestrel
Intrauterine "system" with hormones	Mirena (Schering Brasil)	Intrauterine device (with reservoir containing the hormone levonorgestrel)

Cost/duration	Availability in Salvador
US$18 for a pack of 28	Launched specifically as an extended-regime contraceptive, Elaní contains the hormone drospirenone and is marketed as the "well-being" pill.
US$13 for a pack of 28	Marketed as an extended regime specifically for menstrual disorders.
Varies with cost of individual pills (from US$1 to US$20 for a 21-pill pack); one extra pack of 21 is required for every 3 months of continuous use.	Widely available in public and private health centers or directly over the counter where prescriptions are not always required for purchasing contraceptives. Most of the women interviewed who had used the pill had at one point taken it continuously.
Prices range from US$10 for Depo-Provera to US$5 for Contracep (for a contraceptive efficacy of three months).	Widely distributed method in public health family planning dispensaries and readily available over the counter in pharmacies, many of which apply the injection for a small fee.
Prices range from US$200 to US$900 for a contraceptive efficacy of one to three years, depending on the combination.	Limited to private practices with doctors capacitated to insert the subdermal implants. Common in Salvador because of the active presence of CEPARH, which provides and inserts implants on behalf of other doctors and trains doctors in implant insertion.
US$325 plus medical honorariums. Contraceptive efficacy of three years.	Far less common in Brazil than locally "manipulated" hormonal implants mixing different hormonal compounds.
US$350 plus medical honorariums. Contraceptive efficacy of up to five years.	Limited to private practices because of the high cost. Brazil has the world's highest rate of Mirena use according to several Schering informants.

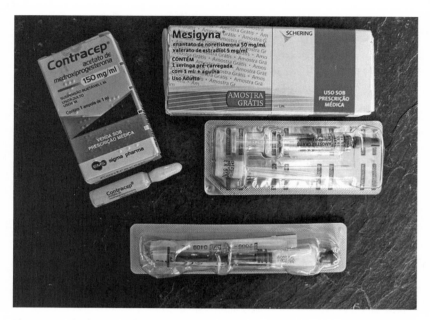

Figure I.5 The hormonal injections most commonly found in Salvador are Depo-Provera's "similar" Contracep (medroxyprogeseterone acetate 150 mg/mL), Depo-Provera, and the monthly injection Mesigyna. Photograph by Emilia Sanabria.

scripts. Interestingly, medical professionals did not always recognize the shared lived experiences widely imputed to sex hormones as hormonally induced. For example, many women experience headaches or weight gain, a fact that was often rebutted by doctors with the refrain: *Hormônio nao engorda, é comida que engorda. Fecha boca, querida* [Hormone doesn't cause weight gain, food does. Close your mouth, darling].

Martin (2006) calls attention to the displacements at work in assessments of pharmaceutical effects. She reviews how adverse side effects are displaced to small print, how population-level effects of clinical trials are off-shored to the developing world, or how marketing and clinical practice keeps the ambivalence people may have about the limited or at times toxic efficacies of the *pharmakon* at bay. While negative effects are laboriously kept "over on 'the side,'" Martin (2006, 282) reminds us that it is "a short step from side effects to 'collateral damage.'" Drawing on Martin's analysis, Masco (2013) asks: "what makes one outcome the benefit of the drug, and another its negative side effect? How is it that this powerful line is drawn, and what forms of value are revealed in its calculus?"[7] The ways in which the potentially harmful effects of sex hormones are assessed and regulated are variable and contested (Löwy and Weisz 2005).[8] A considerable epidemiological literature on the risks of venous thrombosis in oral contraceptives users points to the increased risk for smokers or women using first-generation pills that were more highly dosed.[9] While risks fell with second-generation pill use, controversies resurfaced in the wake of new studies into the increased risks carried by third- and fourth-generation pills, which presented small but consistent increased risks of thrombosis in relation to second-generation pills (see de Bastos et al. 2014; DeLoughery 2011; Marks 2001; and Stegeman et al. 2013 for a discussion of earlier risks).[10] A recent Cochrane review comparing extended-cycle with traditional cyclic dosing (a bleeding interval every three months versus monthly) is curiously contradictory on the topic of safety (Edelman et al. 2014). The widely available abstract states that evidence from randomized controlled trials "is of good quality" and that continuous dosing is "a reasonable approach." But buried in the full-text version one finds the mention, almost in passing, that "the studies were too small to address efficacy, rare adverse events, and safety." My own reading of the data reviewed in this meta-analysis (which includes a 1995 study conducted by Coutinho's team in Salvador) reveals that more than half the studies cited reported conflicts of interest with the pharmaceutical industries whose drugs are trialed. Endocrinologists Prior and Hitchcock (2014) note that with the extended-regime pill, women are exposed to 25–33 percent increased estrogen exposure. A meta-analysis of cardiovascular risks showed that even the pills with the lowest dose cause a doubling of the risk for stroke and heart attack (Baillargeon et al. 2005). Existent studies are biased, Prior and Hitchcock argue, because they compare risks with risks on standard regimen pills and not with untreated menstrual cycles. Further, the continuous pill regimen causes more days of higher-than-normal estrogen concentrations, which is likely to have an incidence on breast cancer.

Depo-Provera, a popular method in my field site, underwent numerous controversies in its career as a contraceptive. The FDA withheld approval for Depo-Provera in 1967, 1978, and 1983 and then approved it in 1992 despite outcry from women's health movements. In 2004, concerns over loss of bone density in Depo-Provera users led the FDA to request a warning highlighting concerns about loss of bone density and indicating that Depo-Provera should not be used for more than two years. Such warnings were absent from the Depo-Provera applications that I observed. In Bahia, risk-benefit analyses put forward the substantial personal and public health consequences of unwanted pregnancies or emphasize the reversibility of long-acting hormonal methods in relation to sterilization—the rates of which are still very high.[11]

I do not engage here in a debate over the relative safety of different hormonal methods, but rather attend to how the potential deleterious effects of hormones are—or are not—raised in Bahia and how these inflect patterns of use. What is most striking about the question of the potential risks associated with hormonal methods is the absence of debate within the Bahian medical community. This was evident both in the interviews I carried out with doctors and in the gynecological conferences I attended. Patients often did raise concerns, but these tended to focus more on experienced side effects rather than concerns with future health risks, such as thrombosis or cancer. These were routinely met with the ready-made, finely tuned, and locally sensitive counterarguments that pharmaceutical sales representatives and doctors establish through their interactions. Oldani (2004) has shown how these ground-level exchanges between pharmaceutical representatives and doctors can inflect local marketing strategies, leading to adjustments in how a pharmaceutical is used and thought about in different prescribing ecologies. In Bahia, I found that doctors' risk–benefit evaluations tended to downplay future health risks in order to ensure compliance and the correct use of hormonal methods in a context where women are seen as switching and swapping erratically, without medical advice. Emphasis was placed on finding the most adapted method, and this often meant bracketing potential health concerns. Women also were engaged in complicated risk–benefit exercises. As I detail in chapter 3, these risk evaluations do not limit themselves to evaluations of health risks. Users' cost–benefit analyses include thinking through the potential costs of not using hormones, which might range from unwanted pregnancy, incapacity to work because of heavy menstrual symptoms, or loss of libido, leading one's husband to stray. Returning to Masco's question concerning how the line between primary and side effect is drawn, we can see the importance of context in shaping how benefits and risks are evaluated. Bahia, with its specific forms of stratified reproduction (Ginsburg and Rapp 1995), has played an important role in the development of the practice of menstrual suppression, that is, in the transmutation of what was initially perceived as a negative side effect of long-acting hormonal methods (the suppression of monthly menstrual episodes) into a desirable end goal. The cloaking of risks in Bahian medical practices should be thought alongside the labor of making evidence about safety for markets in the Global North. They are part of a common regime of value in which lively capital (Sunder Rajan 2012) is produced out of the circulations of pharmaceuticals and their attendant knowledges. Producing new efficacies for sex hormones is facilitated by what Lovell (2006) has aptly termed "pharmaceutical leakage." Leakage describes how pharmaceuticals are shaped by the movements of drugs through global spaces of research, development, production, marketing, and regulation. As sex hormones circulate globally they leak between official and unofficial prescription regimes, reconfiguring bodies and socialities by circulating "not only through blood, brain, and other body sites but also through social settings" (Lovell 2013, 131).

Salvador da Bahia

Over the course of eighteen months, I attended several hundred family planning consultations at CEPARH and in three health posts or maternity units where hormonal contraceptives are dispensed. I interviewed doctors about their work in state-funded services and in their private practices. During participant observation activities in these clinical contexts, I sat in on the stages of *triagem*, observed the preinterview with the nurse and social worker, as well as the consultation itself, during which methods are administered, injected, or inserted. I also went out with CEPARH's municipality-funded mobile unit (CEPARH-móvel) to several *favelas* and partook in a variety of women-centered community activities in these peripheral neighborhoods. Access to gynecological consultations in the private sector was more limited than in the public sector, whose users are presented as appropriate research subjects by medical professionals. My access to the private sector was via the operating theater in two private institutions, where I was able to observe hysteroscopies, laparoscopies, and a dozen births, of which the majority were by cesarean delivery. In CEPARH and in a small neighboring town's maternity unit I was also able to observe three tubal ligations, a dozen vasectomies,[12] and one postabortion curettage. This enabled me to situate hormone use as an engine of new sexual normativities in the changing biopolitical arrangements that link national progress to the constitution of a sexually healthy Brazilian population (Adams and Pigg 2005).

I also conducted over sixty in-depth interviews with women across the class spectrum. These women were urban (although some were of rural origin) and of mixed socioeconomic background. The openness with which

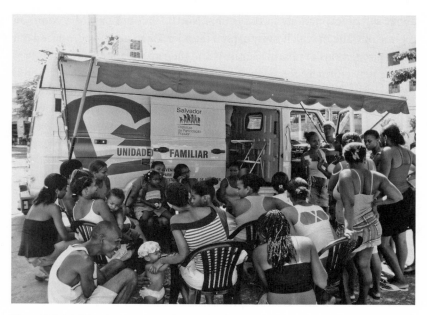

Figure I.6 Waiting for contraceptive methods in the shade of CEPARH's mobile unit in a low-income peripheral neighborhood. Photograph by Emilia Sanabria.

people in Brazil speak publicly about their bodies' most intimate processes has never ceased to amaze me—perhaps the product of having lived in England for so long. Not only are bodies publicly made visible in specific ways, but the women I encountered draw on an array of widely circulated techniques, health tips, pharmaceutical regimens, or physical exercises to modulate their bodies and its processes and to monitor its metamorphoses. I felt my own body scrutinized in particular ways as I entered into clinical spaces where class boundaries are reestablished through close attention to physical appearance, dress, and presentation. But, more importantly, I began to feel differently in my body, to pay attention to things I had never noticed before. Digestion and the specific effects of foods, the embodied manifestations of emotions, the state of one's blood pressure, the relative efficacy of different brands of painkillers, or the reference values for a normal white blood cell count formed part of everyday conversations across a range of social contexts and brought my attention to processes to which I realized I had never given much thought. I was surprised by the extensive knowledge many women had of the different contraceptive methods available, their recommended uses or side effects, and often felt slightly inept when women were surprised to discover that I was quite literally doing exploratory research and not myself always as biomedically versed as they were.

I did not deliberately discriminate between informants in function of sociological categories, speaking to women of diverse backgrounds and with a broad range of views and attitudes toward menstruation and hormones. Within these discussions, I privileged questions about contraceptive choice, experiences of menstruation, reproductive histories, gender relations, and perceived generational shifts in these areas. The topics of sexuality, body culture (narrated to me as a Brazilian specificity), "self-care," medications, well-being, beauty, changing family structure, and abortion regularly arose, demarcating the discursive field within which sex hormone use is commonly situated.[13] During the initial period of fieldwork (2005–6), and in four subsequent visits of three to six months between 2008 and 2013, I attended medical congresses and carried out several weeks of fieldwork in three pharmacies catering to low-, middle-, and high-income neighborhoods. I met pharmacy sector regulators and members of pharmacist professional organizations. I interviewed the national marketing directors of four major pharmaceutical corporations in São Paulo (Schering, Pfizer, Libbs, and Boehringer Ingelheim) and followed the work of Schering's, Libbs's, and Organon's regional managers over the course of several months. I met a number of other pharmaceutical representatives in doctors' waiting rooms, some of whom allowed me to observe their work. Through these contacts I was invited to several pharmaceutical promotion events (such as promotional dinners and in-congress events). Several informants suggested I go to the blood donation center to find answers to my questions about hormônio, blood, and menstruation. There I encountered patients who no longer menstruated and sought to alleviate themselves of the excess blood accumulated by this absence of menstruation (Sanabria 2009, 2011). For several months I also participated in ATRAS's (the Association of Travestis of Salvador) weekly meetings and organized group discussions on travesti uses of hormones. Travestis, as they refer to themselves, are physiological males who use female sex hormones (among other techniques) to transform their bodies. I had not initially anticipated to trace hormones all the way into these sites but, as I detail in chapter 4, this enabled me to understand how hormones are rendered as a kind of substance in Bahia, not unlike blood.

Brazil's first capital and home to a large afro-descendent population, Salvador counts nearly 3 million inhabitants (IBGE 2013). The city spans a vast heterogeneous urban space between the Bay of All Saints, the open sea, and

inland hills. Recent modernization includes the renovation of the old colonial center (*Pelourinho*), the expansion of middle-class neighborhoods along
the seafront, and development of vast tourism installations for both national (Brazilian) and foreign tourists. The Northeast is considered the poor-
est of the five Brazilian macro-regions, wherein wealth is disproportionately
concentrated in Salvador. Despite its size, Salvador has the feel of a small
city, and it is often said that *Salvador é um ovo* (Salvador is an egg) when gossip
gets around with astonishing velocity. Bahia occupies a place that is carefully set apart as sensual, jovial, and backward by Southerners of São Paulo
or Rio. Many have attempted to capture the core elements of this *baianidade*
(Bahian-ity), which, aside from the slurry speak commonly associated by
Paulistas (residents of São Paulo) with the purportedly "lazy" Northeasterner
laborers, includes the specific style of samba (different from that practiced
in Rio), the particular culinary tradition, or Bahian religiosity and "popular culture." Salvador is often characterized by its *sincretismo* (syncretism),
a representation in the national Brazilian imaginary that owes much to the
idea that Brazil is the product of the mixture of the three races: European,
African, and indigenous. The specificities that mark Bahia are often attributed in popular representations to the strong presence of "Africa" in Bahia,
a legacy of slavery. Parés (2006) and van de Port (2011) have noted the importance of the colonial Baroque heritage to Bahian modes of being, suggesting that what is often taken for an African heritage is the product of
a long history of hybridization and mixture that cannot be reduced to the
problematically bounded entities "Africa" or "Europe," as they so often are. I
was in São Paulo in January 2006 when the case of Father Pinto's excommu-
nication from his Catholic parish in Salvador hit the national news. The controversy began during the epiphany celebrations when the priest was said
in the national press to have "turned mass into a show" by staging a celebration to, in his words, "honor the different races of Brazil," representing
each of the three kings as "white," "black," and "Indian." What shocked was
the fact that he appeared in full makeup, emulating an Amerindian dance
and appearing as Oxum, a female Afro-Brazilian deity dressed in gold. Arriving from Bahia, people I met in São Paulo jokingly distanced themselves
from these Bahian extremes of cultural "miscegenation," exclaiming: "Só na
Bahia, né!" (Only in Bahia, no?). Bahians often narrate Bahia as a particularly
"spiritual" place. Among medical professionals I met many Kardecist spi-
ritists, a Christian-based religion founded on the channeling of predominantly eighteenth-century European spirits, a doctrine of reincarnation, and

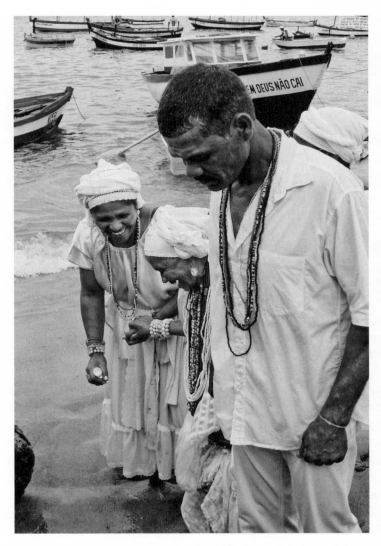

Figure I.7 Two Mães-de-santo (Candomblé priestesses) share a joke at Iemanja festival, Rio Vermelho (Salvador). Photograph by Emilia Sanabria.

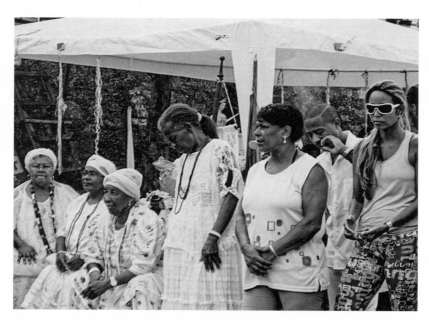

Figure I.8 Bahian "multiculturalism": Candomblé folk and a white middle-class woman observing a ritual dance during Iemanja festival. Photograph by Emilia Sanabria.

healing performed at a distance. A wide array of energy healing practices grew out of this rich polysemous context, and biomedicine is, in a sense, but one of many resources that people call on in their search for health. As Dra Eugenia, a gynecologist I interviewed in her private practice, explained: "Here everything is miscegenation. See that image of the Virgin behind you? That was given to me by Mãe Carmen do Gantois [a well-known Candomblé priestess], and in the bottom corner of the frame is Krishna. Here [shows key ring] is Sai Baba. I love Candomblé, and I like to go to mass at Our Lady of Conceção. You see, I'm Bahian, I'm genuinely ecumenical."

Many have attempted to characterize Brazil's specific sexual culture, emphasizing the sensuality that marks many aspects of sociality and invites "passionate encounters" (Van de Port 2011, 48). Drawing on Freyre's (1990) analysis of sexual miscegenation as foundational to the Brazilian nation, Parker (1991, 28) argued that, in Brazil, sexual life acquired a central importance at the sociocultural level, whereas in Euro-American contexts it is treated as a private or individual phenomenon. In this reading, Brazilian society is heir to the social organization characteristic of the slave-owning *fazenda* (estate). The fazenda connected the patriarch, his wife, and his legitimate offspring to a network of relations that included the patriarch's mistresses, illegitimate children, slaves, tenants, friends, and clients. This, Parker (1991, 31) argues, produced a notion of masculinity tied to the image of the virile and hierarchically superior patriarch and a plural model of femininity, as "legal wife and mother" or "concubine" (5). The different roles of women as objects of desire or as respectable wife and mother are at times difficult to reconcile, and part of what Brazilian feminists denounce as the double standards of sexual morality, whereby male sexuality is encouraged and positively valued, whereas women are expected to elicit desire without compromising their virtue. Parker's analysis is focused almost exclusively on male sexual discourse, allowing him to capture the tenor of *machismo* ideology in a vivid way, using the crude, sexist language of his informants. The extent to which this glorified sexual culture is actually reflected in everyday intimate relations has, however, been questioned (Galvão and Diaz 1999). Drawing on a survey of 4,634 youths in three Brazilian capitals, the authors of the GRAVAD study of young people's sexuality and reproductive trajectories argue that this representation of Brazil as a sexually uninhibited society coexists with a rigid system of gender relations and familial organization that spans all classes (Aquino et al. 2003; Heilborn et al. 2006; Heilborn, Aquino, and Knauth 2006; Heilborn and Cabral 2013). Many of the doctors and health practitioners I spoke with told me that a surprising number of patients consulted for sexual problems. In this context, the capacity attributed to hormones to generate sexual effects—both stimulating desire and protecting from unwanted pregnancy—was particularly appreciated.

When my partner and I first settled in Salvador, we opted for the 2 *de julho* neighborhood, a lower-middle-class, slightly bohemian neighborhood in the old center, lodged between the Campo Grande, the exclusive seafront Vitoria avenue, and *crackolândia* that gentrification and real estate pressure has yet to prevail over. Campo Grande is a central node for many of Salvador's convoluted bus routes. I spent hours negotiating these routes on my way to distant, painstakingly arranged appointments with doctors, health planners, or interviewees who had at times forgotten me by the time I made it to their door. Riding the overpacked, overheated bus up to Federação, where CEPARH is located, one passes steep roads leading into some of the neighborhoods that house the older Candomblé houses of the city.

One spot just after the old cemetery always caught my attention; in the early mornings there would often lie a fresh offering to a *santo* (saint), a yellow ceramic bowl left at the crossroad, the wings of the sacrificial chicken flapping in the morning breeze. One morning I sat behind an ancient little lady who boarded the bus at the large public hospital in Canela. She wore a faded green dress, plastic shoes, and an old stained handkerchief to contain her vibrant white Afro. She carried a battered plastic bag and multitudes of little bags within it, full of treasures, buttons, a shredded identity card, papers that had been folded so many times that it was not clear how they still held together, a single white pill cut out of a blister pack, a little key, a rubber band. She shifted these from one plastic bag back to the other, reorganizing her world. Each of these possessions was manipulated with great care as she knotted and unknotted the little bags and handled these documents, keys into the labyrinthic bureaucracy that I found so challenging to negotiate and that can make citizenship a perpetually receding horizon for many Brazilians. I observed her as we rode down *Barra avenida*, with its Land Rovers; shiny, Lycra-clad, siliconed joggers hooked up to their iPhones; straight, blond, mega-hair extensions; arts cinema; *sorveterias* (ice cream parlors); top-end pharmacies with their imported pharmaceuticals and cosmetics; exclusive diagnostic imagery labs; and *salão de beleza* (beauty parlors), struck by the vivid contrasts so characteristic of Brazilian urban centers.

Over the years I have come to love and long for this city like few other places in the world, despite its intense inequalities, receding public space, and intense commercialism. There is something about the sensuousness and aliveness of Salvador that is hard to capture. A vibrancy in the way I observe my friends engaging in life with joy, letting things unfold even when they struggle with financial difficulties, the absence of the state or the violence that marks the everyday. The strange risk evaluations that shape existence, as one crosses into the peaceful square where seniors gossip, in the early evening freshness, to the monotonous sound of chanting from the mass held on the corner, church doors wide open onto the world, where a shooting occurred in broad daylight, only weeks before, killing three people, one of whom was a pregnant woman. Feral bare-bottomed children play in the ornamental vegetation, their mother lying, disheveled, on a length of cardboard beneath a bench, having visibly made a visit to nearby crackolândia. A huge iguana with sharp teeth observes the scene as two men theatrically exchange a verbal joust, cheered on by onlookers. On one corner a vendor sells pink, blue, and orange popcorn from an antique trolley, topped with

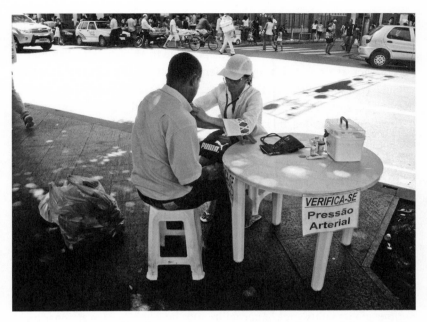

Figure I.9 Measuring blood pressure on a street corner. Photograph by Emilia Sanabria.

condensed milk for an extra *real*. Next to him a coconut water vendor and a corn-on-the-cob vendor are rehearsing the latest carnival hit's suggestive choreography, well aware of the attention their sensual dancing is eliciting. Buses, people, traffic. At the opposite corner a woman in a white lab coat and matching baseball cap has set up a white plastic chair and table and is measuring blood pressure and glucose plasma levels for a small fee. She is a nursing auxiliary and tops up her earnings in this manner. Outside the bank is a good spot to catch hypertension, she jokes, gesturing to the long queue of people waiting to pay bills or renegotiate a loan.

In this book I show that the extreme incursion of biomedical interventions into people's lives in Brazil should be considered alongside other, older, or more mundane forms of bodily management, such as the regular monitoring of blood pressure on a street corner between errands. Bodily processes are of great interest to *Soteropolitanos* (inhabitants of Salvador). Clinical exams of all descriptions—from blood tests to scans, functional magnetic resonance imaging or x-rays—are remarkably present in a context marked by such disparities in access to health care. These imaging techniques constitute a new set of tools to assess, measure, and quantify the bodies' internal metamorphoses. This marked attention to bodies is not limited to the assessments made possible by these medical technologies; rather, their astonishing prevalence attests to the fact that these respond to existing concerns. Dumit (2012, 181–96) has outlined three modes of biomedical living with mass health in the United States. These are "expert patienthood," "fearful subjects," and "better living through chemistry." Here, pharmaceuticals are mobilized to mitigate the risks generated by the new regime of surplus health. The statistical model of mass health is marked by an encroaching paradigm of treatment as prevention in which health and illness are no longer "states of being" (13) but reconfigured as epistemic claims at the population level. This invites patients to become responsible, self-diagnosing experts of their own health, monitoring their blood levels regularly, for example. As Dumit (2012, 192–93) notes, this mode of better (pharmaceutical) living "offers a new choice through reconfiguring what is considered foundational and fixed and what is changeable and can be countered." In Plastic Bodies I examine how biology and nature may also supply notions of instability and changeability and show how human action is often geared to fixing and stabilizing this flux. "Knowing your numbers" in this way takes on a magical quality, enabling expert patients to navigate dysfunctional health systems and make (new) sense of their bodies' changing internal balance.

While characterized by profound inequalities, statistics place Brazil among the highest users of female sterilization, cesarean deliveries, and plastic surgery (Edmonds 2010). The 2002 EngenderHealth publication on female sterilization reported Brazil as having the third highest international rate of female sterilization, placing it above China. Victora et al. (2011) report in The Lancet that 47 percent of all births in Brazil were by cesarean delivery, a rate higher than has been reported in any other country. Cesarean deliveries are performed on 48 percent of primiparous mothers and account for 35 percent of deliveries in the SUS (Sistema Único de Saúde, the public health service), where three-quarters of births take place. The National Agency of Supplementary Health reported in 2008 that 85 percent of births in the Brazilian private health sector were by cesarean delivery, and one of the clinics in which I worked boasted a 99 percent rate. In an article exploring the prevalence of cesarean deliveries in Salvador, McCallum (2005a, 226–27) argues that:

The sexually adapted, attractive and active female body — the proper condition of modern Brazilian women — is represented by untouched and aesthetically pleasing genitalia. These genitalia, if also used for giving birth, lose their power to signify modernity and progress. On the contrary, when sexuality and reproduction become inter-linked through vaginal childbirth, the meanings attached to the genitalia's referent (the female body) are inverted. Such a body is pre-modern, damaged. It is repulsive to others. . . . That this old-fashioned form of birth is also seen as "natural" confers no value on it whatsoever. On the contrary, nature itself is devalued, measured against the gains conferred by science and technology. Abdominal birth lends modernity, and thus continued value, to women's bodies. . . . And women are agents only insofar as they "choose" the knife — and, by this token, "modernity."

The relation between class, modernity, and practices of bodily modification and enhancement therefore needs to be carefully examined. Accounting for the unusually high levels of biomedical interventions solely through the lens of medicalization — that is, the domestication of social inequities with medical solutions that conceal the sociopolitical roots of ill-health (see Scheper-Hughes 1992, for example) — seemed unsatisfactory to me. Throughout fieldwork, in listening to the stories of women who actively sought out such interventions and in observing their engagements with biomedical institutions, procedures, and technologies, it dawned on me that although this was certainly an important part of the story, other things were going on.

Plastic Relations: Class, Race, and Bodies

Dr. Ricardo picked me up at 6 a.m., and we made it to the maternity unit by 7 a.m., at which time a long queue of patients had already formed. The unit was small, making the process of triage explicit, that whole business of counting people, turning their stories into ticked boxes, percentages, and pharmacological formulas. I was numb with that kind of numbness you get when you flick through TV channels and hypnotize yourself. Faces, stories, questions all merged into each other. I had a revelation as I realized that after six hours of attending some fifty patients, all these persons blended into one other, becoming a mass of cases. That experience was an unwitting moment of participation in what is often referred to in Bahia as the "dehumanization" of medical attention. It was the point at which my under-standing of medical practice shifted and came to include an understanding of how things felt for doctors in this context of scarce resources and the "social problem," as Ricardo refers to it. We walked down a corridor, to the "private" part of the unit, newly built and latched onto the old crumbling pink colonial building. Several neatly dressed patients were waiting. He exchanged caring words, hugs, kisses, and jokes with them. We took place in the very new, air-conditioned *consultório*, where there was markedly more time for listening and discussing, more space for negotiation, for finding a way (*dar jeito*). The contrast, so proximate, was striking. Most of the gyne-cologists I met juggled several jobs, moving on the same day from the private to the public sector (SUS).[14] The typical pattern is attending patients in a SUS health post or public maternity hospital in the morning and holding private consultations in the afternoon.

We had a quick lunch in the hospital cafeteria, and idle talk rapidly gave way to sexist jokes exchanged between the hospital's director, Mineiro the anesthetist (a self-proclaimed *petista* [PT activist] studying for a law degree), and Ricardo. After a phenomenally sweet but much needed coffee, we went straight up to the labor ward where four young, heavily pregnant women awaited "their [scheduled] surgeries." We proceeded into the operating theater for the first delivery. I was impressed by how quick it was: twenty-seven minutes from the first incision to the final stitch. The baby was whisked off by the pediatric nurse and we moved on to the next surgery in the neighbor-ing, posher, and newer private operating theater. The second baby was extracted. We moved back into the first, which had been cleaned up and where patient number three lay waiting. Everything stood out starkly with the other room: the electrosurgical scalpel was Cellotaped together, although it might now be considered a piece of 1950s design, the operating table was rusty at the edges, and so on. The surgical protocol swung into action, but this time things didn't go smoothly. The baby was fine but the patient stirred, and Mineiro kept having to leave his law books to increase the dose of anesthetic. Tension rose. He and Ricardo exchanged stern words: "you deal with your bit and leave the head to me [*deixa a cabeça comigo*]," Mineiro re-torted. Joking ceased. There was profuse bleeding and Ricardo and the nurse worked, silent, highly focused, their shoes splattered with birth blood. Time dragged on, but the situation had come under control by the time the direc-tor popped his head through the door and asked what on earth was going on. Ricardo turned away from the operating table, exposing a long flow of blood that had stained his overalls from the crotch down. Catching sight of this, Mineiro burst out laughing and pointing to the blood exclaimed: "The patient started to whine and moan and *Ricardinho* got so emotional that he menstruated [*fico menstruado*]!"

Roughly 75 percent of Soteropolitanos rely on the SUS (the national health service), which operates according to the principles of universality of services, equality of all citizens, and integration of health actions. Founded in 1988, the SUS still faces major challenges and is marked by lack of resources, leading those who can afford it to take out a *plano de saúde* (medical insurance). Twenty-five percent of the population has private health insurance, which gives them access to a range of services, including highly sophisticated, top-of-the-range medical services. Doctors, clinics, hospitals, and clinical laboratories have *convênios* (agreements) with different *planos*. These vary widely in the services they cover, the clinics they give access to, and so on, compounding the stratification between "private" and "public" health even further.[15] At one extreme, state-funded services vary (some are indeed excellent), but are generally characterized by lack of resources and long queues. In a context of stretched resources and overwhelming demand, the question of *atendimento* (medical attention) is intrinsically tied up with discussions concerning *cidadania* (citizenship) in a context where the right to health is still very much in the making (Biehl and Petryna 2013). Medical practices and pharmaceutical drugs are used to fulfill societal expectations of work, appropriate fertility, and beauty, and to signal new social relations. Given that the range of possibilities extends unevenly from very little access to health care to high-tech, specialist-led medical intervention, with little in between, both possibilities become charged with particular values. I became interested in how people in Salvador adopt medical technologies, in a context marked, on the one hand, by the problem of overmedication and a predilection for surgical operations, and by an absence of quality primary care on the other. Medicine is a highly significant social institution in the making of urban Brazilian identities in a context where the highly differentiated class structure is reflected in access to health care (Barbosa et al. 2002; Biehl 2004, 2005; Corrêa 2001; Edmonds 2007, 2010; McCallum 2005a; Scheper-Hughes 1992). McCallum (2005a) suggests that health insurance itself functions as a marker of class distinction.

The protests that took place across Brazil in June 2013 exposed massive popular unrest over the limits of public services such as health care. The economic boom of the 1990s and 2000s, which gave Brazil a new standing as no longer the "country of the future" — as Brazilians commonly say — but an "emergent nation" and key player on the international scene (Pinheiro-Machado and Dent 2013), left many behind as deep inequalities persisted. Aquino (2014) argues that the protests exposed the fact that the SUS is unable to ensure quality services to all, noting that the 25 percent of Brazilians who have private health insurance benefit from tax waivers, which effectively finances with public money the access to private care for this privileged minority. At stake here are contrasting visions of public health in a context where the health system's shortcomings are often glossed over as technical problems or problems of resources, when they are also — and at times primarily — political (Aquino 2014). Many Brazilian feminist scholars of health note the current de-politicization of health issues in relation to the radicalness and comprehensiveness with which public health was rethought in the post-military transition of the 1980s (Aquino 2014; Costa 2009; Diniz 2012). Diniz (2012, 126) notes that the inclusion of the social and political aspects of health in the Women's Comprehensive Health Care Program (PAISM), launched in 1983, "lost ground to the discourse of access to medical consumption." Likewise, Aquino (2014) and Diniz (2012) note policy back-peddling over the achievements that were conquered under PAISM, most notably from religious and conservative lobbies.[16]

The period 1945–1980 saw massive changes in urban Brazilian class structures following rapid industrialization. Gender, work relations, and attitudes to leisure, the body, and health shifted dramatically as women entered paid employment. In their history of urban class formation, Mello and Novais (1998) explain that industrialization enabled the ascension into the middle classes of a new class of unskilled workers such as sales assistants or low-paid office clerks. Given the legacy of slavery and the perpetuation of a "culture of servitude," physical labor lies at the bottom of the hierarchy of employment and is stigmatized among the middle classes. Work is evaluated according to the degree of (dis)pleasure it affords, and distinctions are made between work that is clean or dirty, light or heavy, routine or creative, subaltern or managerial, and the years of formal education required to enter into a profession. Upward stratification produced a new class of managers, the rise of a service industry (publicity agencies, market research companies, etc.), and with it a new professional elite who joined the traditional elite (comprising doctors, lawyers, landowners, and businessmen). The "stressed out bodies and tormented minds" of this new class of professionals were — as Mello and Novais (1998, 629) impart, not without irony—in turn attended to by a growing body of psychoanalysts, astrologists, cardiologists, plastic surgeons, entertainment promoters, gym owners, divorce lawyers, massage therapists, interior decorators, endocrinologists, dermatologists, and others. The success of these specialties in Brazil is accounted for by reference to a process of "moralization," which challenges the authority of the church, upholding in its place ideals of *aperfeiçoamento* (self-improvement) through work, spiritual development, and hygiene. This link between work, hygiene, and class is central to contemporary Brazilian class relations. A brief overview of the historical formation of these ideas reveals how the hygienist movement produced the body as a site of intervention. In the early twentieth century concerns with hygiene and propriety came to occupy a central role in processes of social differentiation and class. Physical and moral education were seen as necessary to the project of producing healthy bodies, contained, polite individuals, demarcating the *culto* (cultivated) from the *inculto* (ignorant). The Brazilian historian Jurandir Freire Costa (2004) argued that this produced *higiene* as "emblematic of social differentiation," a mark of class that distinguishes *senhores* (gentry) from their subalterns. This movement of hygienic control transformed the "colonial family" by supplanting religious and patriarchal codes of conduct with an infinitely variable hygienic—and, increasingly, an esthetic—one (see Edmonds 2013). Some of the women I interviewed achieved what one might refer to as "middle-class status" through work or marriage, and their reproductive trajectories and bodily projects are marked by this class transition.[17]

The minute details of physical appearance are carefully monitored and Soteropolitanos are able to deduce a great deal about a person's social status by analyzing their appearance, the neatness, style, and quality of their clothes and shoes, as well as their gait and demeanor. Access to employment is contingent on *boa aparencia* (good appearance), a criterion that blends beauty, presentation, locution, and *jeito* (manner/bodily expression). Although the economic means of achieving boa aparencia are unevenly distributed, beauty and bodily care are important means of social ascent, rendering bodies sites where social hierarchies are renegotiated. The *interior* (rural zones) remains an important category of alterity in Brazil and often serves as a narrative foil to explain the substantial changes that have taken place in urban Brazilian society. Crucial to this process of differentiation is the concept of modernity, as implicit in the idea that people from the interior are *atrasados* (behind), or still hold to backward or ignorant traditional beliefs. On one occasion, my partner, young daughter, and I returned to Salvador after a weekend break. We opted to travel by the *barco de nativos* (literally, "the native's boat") rather than the speedboat most middle-class beachgoers use. At 5 a.m., an old tractor wove its way along the single village road, picking up passengers. Sleeping children were gently passed into the tightly packed rows of passengers on the hard wooden bench, along with luggage, sacks of produce, and baskets enclosing chickens. At around 6 a.m. we arrived at a small river port and embarked upon a two-hour journey to Valença, a small town a few hours' bus journey from Salvador. We boarded silently and took advantage of the boat's rocking motion to gain a little more rest. Then suddenly, obeying a signal unbeknownst to us, the boat awoke to a kind of organized agitation. Hair nets were removed and locks delicately unraveled, children's hair was vehemently combed into order, elaborate makeup was applied, layers of warm clothing to ward off the dawn cool were stripped off, revealing carefully chosen color-coordinated outfits, plastic imitation *havaianas* were swapped for pristine trainers or high-heeled shoes conjured out of bags. As the boat strenuously tugged along the last curve into Valença's port, we observed the astonishing transformation that had taken place among our fellow passengers. While we had initially stood out as a family when we boarded the tractor, we now felt underdressed and disheveled as we entered town. This anecdote brought home to us the considerable importance given to appearance and the intense issues at stake in how one presents as one moves from the interior to the *cidade* (city).

Race is rarely the explicit language people adopt to speak about the "social differences" at work in relations to medical institutions and bodily transformation projects in Bahia.[18] I carried out this research over the course of Luiz Inácio Lula da Silva's two presidential mandates, when large-scale social programs targeting poverty were radically reconfiguring class relations.[19] In the course of my discussions concerning contraceptive options, the salient issues that arose concerned shifting demands on public services, often couched in terms of debates about citizenship and responsibilities and framed within an aspirational politics driven by a desire to consume elite services and goods. In her discussion of race and class in Salvador, McCallum (2005b) takes issue with the emphasis on community-based ethnography in Brazilian anthropology, pointing to the difficulties arising from studying class without founding the discussion on direct observation of cross-class *interactions*. While she is careful to note that in Salvador, the body itself is not the sole or determining basis upon which racial categorizations are made (these also include dress, behavior, locality, and so on), she concedes that bodily differences become imbued with particular—racialized—meanings. But this body is neither finished nor closed and is always the site of production and transformation: "changing its form and meaning, whether through spiritual or magical technological intervention, through diet and exercise, or by medical means" (111). McCallum concludes that although the racialization of bodies is fixed through the repeated re-inscription in spaces and interactions that naturalize class differences, these are contested, wittingly and unwittingly, by changes in the repeated patterns of movements and subjectivity formations, which (re)structures these social hierarchies (113). What I wish to highlight is, notwithstanding the staggering inequities that prevail, the relative malleability and plasticity of identities and the role of bodily transformation therein.

During one of the births that I attended, a fleeting example of the ensuing negotiation between class, race, age, and status caught my attention. The birthing mother was a twenty-three-year-old black woman who worked for a telemarketing company that provided its 90 percent female workforce with medical insurance. Throughout the birth, she resisted the expedient manner with which the medical team sought to see her through her labor, different, I noted, from the way the same team treated women on different health plans. The obstetrical nurse, a stern woman in her early fifties, was highly unsympathetic to the extreme discomfort the birthing mother was in and coldly requested her to turn on her side in order to apply the epidural. The young mother requested assistance, which was met with dry responses of the kind, "If you don't help me I cannot apply the anesthetic to help you." Shifting to her side with great difficulty, in tears, she implored, "O moça, me ajude!" (Oh "girl," please help me!) The nurse flinched, clearly offended by the subtle role reversal this request implied. Within the hierarchies of status in Salvador, it is very common for a young—usually white—person to address an older but socially inferior—usually black—person (e.g., a waiter, shop attendant, cleaner, or taxi driver) by the term moço or moça, which literally means "boy" or "girl." By calling the older, white, and professionally senior nurse moça, this patient was renegotiating the terms of her relationship with the nurse in a manner that implied she was there to serve or assist her. This example illustrates the manner in which class, race, age, status, and the hierarchies they produce are deeply enmeshed and subject to subtle dynamics in the context of shifting social relations.

Weismantel and Eisenman (1998) demonstrate the ways in which race in the Ecuadorian Andes is experienced as both somatic but not biological in origin. Race can be changed over time and yet is embodied. It is "neither genetic nor symbolic, but organic: a constant, physical process of interaction between living things" (Weismantel 2001, 266).[20] Race, Weismantel and Eisenman (1998) argue, accumulates in bodies, in its orifices, organs, impulses, or gait, acquired slowly over a lifetime. The authors note that both the defenders of a biological basis of race and their social-constructivist opponents curiously do not engage with the physicality of bodies, either through a form of antimaterialism that views race as socially constructed, or—where biological racism is concerned—by taking race as genetically determined and "disdaining the natural history of the body after conception" (134). Against such problematic distinctions, they present Andean notions of race as transformative and malleable, arguing that "it is possible to become what one was not at birth" (135) by slowly building a different body.

Historian of science López Beltrán (2007) shows the important role that humoral, Hippocratic ideas about blood played in colonial Latin American racial categories. Blood, in this period, did not lend itself to the kind of biological determinism it would acquire later through the eighteenth and nineteenth centuries. Instead, the humoral notions of blood that prevailed in the colonial and early postcolonial periods could be "diluted, equilibrated, or modified by adequate sets of circumstances. There is no hereditary fatalism in this early period" (272). In sum, social work—such as dress, demeanor, or education—was, and to some extent continues to be, read as having somatic effects. This Hippocratic body is somewhat plastic to its environment. While some features are more tenaciously engrained in the soma, others are open to change—a change that could be transmitted. These historical and Andean foils illustrate the importance that transformations of bodily appearance and countenance can have in subtly reworking social hierarchies. Brazilian anthropologist Mirian Goldenberg (2002, 9) argues that the body has become a kind of capital, and that a well-presented body is seen as a token of one's personal success. Brazilian esthetic practices become a means of social mobility. Likewise, Edmonds (2007, 2010) argues that the beautified body is intimately tied up to and reflects the ambiguous emancipatory power of capital itself in that beauty challenges traditional hierarchies: "Beauty . . . is an unfair hierarchy, but one which can disturb other unfair hierarchies" (2007, 377). As DaMatta (1987) has argued, the passage from casa (house)—hierarchical domain of affect and "personalism"—to rua (street), the domain of impersonal relations between individuals, is ritually marked by the preparation of the body, its dress and presentation, such that personalistic casa hierarchies are maintained in the rua. Increasingly, as Malysse (2002) and Edmonds (2007, 2010) show, bodywork has become a privileged site through which status is renegotiated. Malysse extends the Bourdieusian notion of distinction to the body itself: "the 'natural' body has become synonymous to the poor, or popular body.... Thus, many dream of changing their bodies in order to change classes" (102–3, my translation). What is valued is the energy that each "individual" deploys to (re)construct her identity and to bring her body under control. "Attractiveness has a social effect that seems to short-circuit other networks of power," Edmonds (2010, 17) argues in his analysis of the disproportionate appeal of plastic surgery in Brazil. The growing access to medical services and the relative democratization of health have played an important role in these shifting social hierarchies.

Plasticity and the Borderlands of the Body

Brazilian feminists have been vocal in denouncing the disproportionate encroachment of medicine on all aspects of women's lives and bodies. In a booklet published by the feminist organization Sempreviva, the risks of the imposition of "excessive medicalization and abusive technological intervention on women's bodies" (Faria and Silveira 2000, ii) are highlighted. The authors denounce the normative version of femininity harbored through what they see as medicine's emphasis on youth, beauty, and well-being, arguing this is essentially market-driven rather than aimed at gynecological concerns of greater epidemiological importance to women (such as abortion or access to primary care). Similarly, in a critical essay on "medical intervention" and women's bodies, Rotania (2000), the director of Ser Mulher, an important Brazilian women's nongovernmental organization, denounces interventionism. Rotania deconstructs the discursive logic of the technological cycle within which Brazilian reproductive medicine is embroiled. Her conclusion is that the body has lost its ontological integrity in the face of the ever deeper incursion of medical technologies. This leads her to ask: "If one of the constitutive principles of the concept of reproductive rights is bodily integrity, what kind of rereading is necessary?" (23). Brazilian anthropologist Teresa Caldeira (2000) proposes that in Brazil, the body is "unbounded." She shows how interventions on bodies are perceived as both natural and desirable. The notion of an unbounded body is developed first and foremost to evoke the ways the urban middle classes speak of the bodies of prisoners and criminals. However, in the conclusion to *City of Walls*, she proposes that to understand Brazilian forms of democracy, citizenship, and power it is essential to turn to the micropolitical interactions surrounding bodies. The two specific examples that she proposes will yield further understanding of the problem of violence in Brazil are the domains of "open sensuality" (such as carnival) and the practices of reproductive health, centering on women's bodies. My work begins where hers concludes, as it were. Echoing Rotania's concerns, Caldeira asks whether the respect for individuality and human rights can be imagined for Brazil, where "the body is not respected in its individual enclosure and privacy." For Caldeira, civil rights "depend on the bounding of the body and the individual, and on the recognition of their integrity" (372). What is needed, I propose, is a critical engagement with the notion of the bounded body, which remains the problematic basis upon which Caldeira and others concerned with the violence that characterizes Brazilian social life pin their hopes. While Caldeira's argument is very important, her notion of the "unbounded" body rests on the prior assumption of a bounded body. What is perhaps most problematic about such notions of boundedness is the implicit naturalness upon which they often rest. It is not the unnaturalness of biomedical interventions that should absorb our critical efforts, as so often they do, but their politics.

Plastic Bodies therefore critically engages with notions of bodily integrity and proposes a frame with which to trace how people oscillate between imagining the body as bounded while simultaneously recognizing its malleability. Both positions rest on each other, for conceiving of unboundedness rests on the prior bounding of the body and vice versa. By intervening one is restoring the body to its original state, but this original state is achieved only through intervention. Menstrual suppression is based on a paradoxical proposition: The practice aims to stabilize bodies while inherently assuming their malleability. Menstruation is constructed as a form of bodily instability and hormones as key agents in restoring balance and control. Building on this case, I propose that the stability of the body cannot be assumed here and that constant effort is required to hold it together in the form widely recognized as "the" body. Women who practice menstrual suppression, and doctors who recommend it, deploy various explanatory strategies to rationalize this intervention, drawing on the now familiar and recurrent repertoire of technologizing nature and naturalizing technology (Strathern 1992b). The manner in which bodies are rendered intervenable in

Bahia—their specific local malleability and plasticity—at times resonates with the biomedical version of the body as given and coherent, while continually challenging and re-mapping its limits. Within anthropological approaches, the modern Western body often served as an implicit foil through which local bodily ontologies were revealed. While attesting to the many possible forms of embodiment, both historically and cross-culturally, such approaches at times reinforced the self-evident character the bounded, unitary, Western body was seen to have, or to overly state the fluidity of "exotic" bodily ontologies. As medical anthropologists turned their gaze inward and took up the challenges laid out by science and technology studies to consider scientific and biomedical ontologies as constructed through practices, biology ceased to be perceived as a universal yardstick (Franklin and Lock 2003; Franklin and Ragoné 1998; Haraway 1989, 1991, 1997; Lock 1993; Martin 1994, 2001; Mol 2002; Rapp 2000; Strathern 1992b).

In this book my aim is not to argue that Bahian bodies are plastic while Euro-American ones are stable and fixed. I do not attribute a particular kind of bodily ontology to Bahians as counter-distinct from a purportedly "Western" one.[21] Nor do I map differences between bodily ontologies onto differences *within* Brazil (whether differences of class or ethnicity).[22] Rather, I propose that within the field of hormonal practices described here, one finds both positions simultaneously. Ontologies, Mol (2002) taught us, can be multiple without being exclusive, that is, without relativizing the things to which they refer. Viveiros de Castro and Goldman (2012) argue that confusing multiplicity with relativism is one of anthropology's bad habits. It stems from an understanding of the multiple as that which is opposed to the one. Yet this relation need not be binary, as Haraway (2004, 35) taught us: "One is too few, but two are too many." *Plastic Bodies* attends in an ethnographically engaged manner to the minutia of how bodies (not "the" body) are remade. I read bodies, in their multiple local instantiations, as ongoing and collective materializations.[23] This book examines how sex hormones are enrolled to modulate, transform, and manage women's bodies. I analyze the ways in which sex hormones are consumed—as in literally absorbed, or swallowed—from the perspective of the bodies that absorb them and are modified through them. I take inspiration from Lock and Farquhar's (2007, 1–16) call for a renewed analysis of embodiment in anthropology that addresses the "materialism of lived bodies" and takes us beyond the study of the "body proper." The ethnographic materials presented reveal the way biomedical and social practices surrounding women's leaky and volatile (Grosz

1994) bodies produce bodies as "boundary projects" (Haraway 1991, 200). Considering such "boundary projects" from the perspective of what it means to hold the body stable and to enact its multiplicity as unitary (Mol 2002) or from the perspective of how *removing* things from bodies produces bodies as bounded entities (Kristeva 1982; Weiner 1995), the book gives an ethnographic account of how bodies are (re)made. To do this, I draw on Ingold's (2007, 2010) attempt to rethink phenomenology. Bodies breathe, grow, decay, and their existence depends on their ability to incorporate their environments through the acquisition of skills or nourishment that travel across their ever-emergent surfaces. My aim in engaging with the literatures on bodies and materialities is to think about the relationalities between things that are not clearly or neatly pre-bounded (bodies, on one side, and "things" like pharmaceutical hormones, on the other). The problem I want to address is that of "absorption" in its literal sense of how something material that is not the body becomes the body, acting through it. I highlight the contingent and fragile nature of these objects that are still often taken for bounded in anthropological theory. The book critically engages with the anthropological literature on pharmaceuticals (Petryna, Lakoff, and Kleinman 2006; Whyte, van der Geest, and Hardon 2002) from the perspective of its tendency to take the object for granted, and to not attend to the absorption, dissolution, or enmeshment of the thing into the bodies in which they become efficacious. It shifts the focus from the finished pharmaceutical object to the chemical materials that constitute it, unpacking some of the work that goes into making the bounded object look so solid. As Nading (2014) has argued, chemicals are "ontological engines": tools that humans use to remake life forms, by killing or dulling reproductive capacities, or realign human-microbial assemblages. But they are also "theory machines" that help us rethink the relations between what Idhe (2000) called embodied being and environing worlds.

In this book, I draw on the notion of plasticity, which refers to the capacity to both receive and give form. The definition of *plastic* points simultaneously to the malleability of matter (its capacity to receive form) and to its resistance (the constraints afforded by its existing form). Further, the term *plasticity* holds the potential of troubling any natural referent that might still be associated with the notion of "the body." French philosopher Catherine Malabou has argued for the importance of marking a radical distinction between flexibility on the one hand and plasticity on the other. Flexibility, she argues, implies infinite extendability and polymorphism, and as such it is only one aspect of plasticity (Malabou 2011; Butler and Malabou 2010). To be flexible is to receive form and to yield to constraint in a docile manner. The concept of flexibility lacks the creative potential of giving form: "Flexibility is plasticity minus its genius" (Malabou 2011, 57, my translation). Malabou pins considerable political hopes on the notion of plasticity, thus distinguished from flexibility, which she, as others before her (most notably Martin 1994), suggests has been colonized by neoliberalism. She proposes that plasticity is flexibility's "consciousness to come" (Malabou 2011, 56). Plasticity, thus defined, is open-ended; it has the aptitude to transform destiny, to inflect its form and not just constitute it (65). The polysemous dimensions of the term *plasticity* give it the capacity to bring together two otherwise polarized meanings: that of necessity or determination of form and that of liberty or capacity to become otherwise. The tension between them is what constitutes the force of this concept. My aim is to weave together several aspects of bodily plasticity. First, I attend to the ways bodies are experienced as in flux through an in-depth analysis of how the menstrual cycle is lived as a form of corporeal instability or intrinsic plasticity. Here I draw on Martin's (2001) seminal work on the intersections between women's experiences and medical constructions of the cyclical female body, examining the specific permutations these intersections take on in the Bahian context. Second, I explore the hormonal interventions that are carried out on bodies to modulate and transform them. Engaging with the expansive literature on bodily projects in Latin America, I argue that the recognition and appropriation of bodily plasticity is an integral aspect to the myriad forms through which social hierarchies of race, class, or gender are renegotiated there. I situate hormone use within the frame of other biomedical interventions such as the high rates of cesarean deliveries (McCallum 2005a; Padua et al. 2010; Victora et al. 2011); plastic surgery (Edmonds 2010; Edmonds and Sanabria 2014; Taussig 2012); hysterectomy (Araújo and Aquino 2003); or bariatric surgery.[24] This enables me to provide an account of the significant role ideas about bodies and their transformation play in accounting for the extensive biomedicalization of Brazilian social life.

CHAPTER 1

MANAGING THE INSIDE, OUT

MENSTRUAL BLOOD AND BODILY DYS-APPEARANCE

Menstruation is, in many ways, a banal and unexceptional experience shared by women worldwide. Given that cultural attitudes toward menstruation vary widely, shaping individual women's feelings about the experience in innumerable ways, it is difficult to speak about menstruation per se. Because it is often understood to be, along with pregnancy and childbirth, a defining aspect of womanhood, much of the academic attention it has received pertains to the symbolic role it plays in gender hierarchies (Godelier 1982; Gregor and Tuzin 2001; Héritier 1996; Lewis 1988; Reeves Sanday 1981). In this literature the meanings of menstruation tend to be presented in binary terms as either negative (such as in the case of so-called menstrual pollution beliefs) or positive or in a manner that, in the end, dissociates menstrual symbolism from the physiological process of menstruation. Such analyses tell us relatively little about how women actually experience menstruation.

Drawing on extensive interviews carried out with over sixty women of different social backgrounds in Salvador, I show how menstruation can be at once eagerly anticipated and detested, painful and yet welcome, or considered mucky and nevertheless cleansing. It is precisely these ambiguous aspects of menstruation that I aim to foreground in this chapter. Regardless of whether the women I encountered spoke positively or not of their periods, their experiences of the menstrual cycle reveal that menstruating is often perceived as unsettling a state of normal embodiment. Narratives of menstruation reveal that the experience of cyclicity—however common—is taken as a somewhat exceptional bodily state. Women regularly speak of the emotional and physical changes associated with the menstrual cycle as disrupting their normal sense of self and their usual relationship to their body. Although women spend more time not menstruating than they do menstruating, menstruation is by no means a rare occurrence (as childbirth or serious illness may be). My aim in this chapter is to explore how menstruation can be seen as both a habitual and an exceptional phenomenon. Narratives of menstruation, which posit the body as changeable and at times out of one's control, allow an alternative image of embodiment to emerge. They produce a foil of sorts and are an occasion for the formalization of what—against the posited abnormality of the menstruating body—is taken as normal embodiment. In this chapter I examine the multiple, contradictory, and ambivalent ideas that surround menstrual blood and suggest that concerns regarding menstrual blood serve to manage and delimit bodily orifices. The interviews I conducted with women regarding their experiences of menstruation reveal a surprising degree of bodily awareness and attention to the subtle intricacies of the changes that take place within their bodies. These narratives show that many women have appropriated and given meaning to the myriad symptoms attributed to the hormonal fluctuations of the cycle. While they come to know their bodies in particular ways, this knowledge at times leads them to experience their body as if it were something other than "them." The things that their bodies do are narrated as things that happen to them and that they struggle to reconcile to their selves. In this sense, visceral signals can intercede in the normal relation a person has established with her body, transforming her subjective experience. What implications might this have for the notion of bodily plasticity? My concern here is with the dynamic interplay operating between the body's interiority and its exterior. In the first section of this chapter I examine this relationship through an analysis of how the body's interior processes are made amenable to conscious control. In the second I explore how the management of menstrual blood and the hygienic practices that surround it highlight concerns with policing and, I argue, producing the boundary between the inside and outside of bodies.

Menstruation and Bodily *Dys*-Appearance

In narrating the physical and emotional fluctuations they underwent throughout their menstrual cycles, some of the women I encountered explicitly voiced incertitude concerning the status of what they called their *eu* (me). Such narratives reveal how women attempt to deal with what we might call disjunctions of the self, that is, how they deal with the angry, depressed, or *nervosa* part of themselves that cyclically emerges as a result of hormonal fluctuations. What is striking is the way in which one aspect of the self or bodily experience is taken to be "me" (eu) and others excluded. This has an important social dimension, in that certain aspects of experience are largely excluded, repressed, or otherwise marked as inappropriate by social rules.

None of the women I interviewed was currently using a chart to monitor her cycle, although a few women had done so at one time.[1] However, bodily cues marking different stages of the menstrual cycle were widely reported. Lana, a young woman working as a sales assistant in a clothing store in the popular neighborhood of Piedade, explained in an interview that she did not count the days of her cycle, but always knew when her menstruation was coming as "she" signaled her arrival clearly: "For me, the signal that she is coming is that my breasts are swollen, I get a secretion in my underwear, and a distinctive smell, a bit acidic, you know?" Pricilla, a forty-four-year-old orthodontist and mother of two, uses hormonal implants to suppress her menstrual cycle because she found menstrual cycling challenging:

> My cycle is well defined. I feel ovulation. The difference between the phases is very clear: until ovulation is one phase, I'm *arisca* [horny], and then I feel the day of ovulation. After I ovulate, the "fire" lessens, and then there is another peak just before menstruation. But I feel a lot of alteration. That's why I use the [menstrual suppressive] implant now. The *transtornos* [disruptions] of premenstrual tension were just too much. It gave me a lot of *nervosismo*, I would become a "[tyrannosaurus] rex," it disturbed [things] at home, at work, I was very irritable, impatient, I had pains in my body, I was tired, and then on top of that I would menstruate. It was horrible.

It is interesting to note that the positively valued changes associated with ovulation are expressed in the present tense in Pricilla's narrative, despite the fact that she no longer ovulated at the time of the interview. If anything, this reveals the extent to which, notwithstanding the pharmacological intervention adopted, the baseline state for the female body is to be marked by cyclicity. Aside from being marked by monthly cyclical phases, menstruation changes through the different phases of a woman's life, from menarche to menopause. Many women speak of being "very regular" while giving details of substantial variations in cycle length at different moments in their lives. "Sometimes my cycle can be 32, 35 days with long heavy periods, but at the moment it comes every 25 or 26 days and stays only 3 or 4 days," explains Gabriela, a doctoral student I interviewed. Tatiana, a communication analyst for a state administration, clearly identified distinct phases in her life throughout which her menstrual cycle had evolved. She describes herself as "conscious" of her body, a fact that derives from her "addiction" to yoga—as she qualified it—and her ecumenical spirituality, which draws as much from Candomblé as it does from New Age practices.

Well, the thing is, there are phases in which your menstruation changes. During adolescence, on the first day it would start with a little stain, and then it would come more strongly, proper blood, you know. I didn't pay much attention to it then; I didn't have any symptoms. After, when I was 15–16, I started getting really bad period cramps when my menstruation came down. It would come down all at once and stop very rapidly. Then it got more regular, because it used to drag on for 10 days, starting and ending with that stain. I didn't use to count the days, I only started counting when I took the pill. The pill made it regular, my period became more controlled. Then I stopped the pill, about 2 years ago, and I started to feel when she would arrive, to feel the premenstrual tension. I stopped the pill because it interfered in my sexual desire, and I didn't like it, it gave me the sensation that it wasn't good for me. Now she [menstruation] is in a new phase, I observe myself more. I get irritated. Now my menstruation has come to be like this: I get a cramp the first day, and a headache and pain in my lower back, during the bleeding. I feel symptoms of irritation two days before. That makes me think: "Ah! It's my menstruation! I'm not such a pain."

Detailed analyses of the many transformations occurring throughout the menstrual cycle are common, often centering on the premenstruum. Such narratives tend to present the premenstrual self in ambivalent terms, as other. Here, Tatiana expresses relief when her menstrual blood arrives, allowing her to reinterpret previous ill-humor and to differentiate between the hormonally altered being to which women often allude and her true self.

My question in what follows concerns how certain bodily experiences come to be read as self, whereas others are marked as abnormal or other. How are we to understand the fact that menstruation, a common, repetitive corporeal experience in the lives of many women, nevertheless comes to be marked as an exceptional or abnormal bodily state?

The philosopher Drew Leder (1990) proposes a model to account for the disjunction between the lived body and the self. Leder proposes that Cartesian dualism is in part grounded in bodily experience, a fact that, he argues, accounts for the tenaciousness of mind–body distinctions within and beyond Western culture. He argues that the general mode of embodiment is one in which the body is absent. In the everyday, interactive experience of the body—which he refers to as "ecstatic" corporeality—the body disappears as it is turned onto the world. Ecstatic corporeality is contrasted in his model to bodily *dys*-appearance, the process where, in injury or illness, the body is foregrounded in our experience. When the body dys-appears, the otherwise taken-for-granted body is drawn "out of self concealment," emerging as "an alien presence" (76). He distinguishes between surface and depth disappearance, arguing that the inner or viscous body is even more elusive than the surface, ecstatic body. A viscus, he argues, cannot be "summoned for personal use, turned ecstatically onto the world" (5), as a surface organ may be: "I cannot act from my inner organs in the way I do from my surface musculature. Though I can lift my arm without any problem, I cannot in the same way choose to secrete a little more bile or accelerate my digestion. The 'magical' sway I have over my own body that Merleau-Ponty describes thus refers primarily to the body surface. The depths involve an even deeper sorcery extending beyond my domain" (48).

Citing Ricoeur's reflections on the voluntary and the involuntary and the fact that "life functions in me, without me" (Leder 1990, 46), Leder proposes that it follows that the subject ("I," in his text) experiences this disappearing visceral body as other, as an object. Can Leder's approach be drawn on to explain why the women I encountered often spoke of the body during or before menstruation as different from their self? The notion of dys-appearance is useful here because it highlights the tension that exists between what is taken as normal embodiment (an absence of the visceral body from experience) and the eruption of the visceral in everyday experience. In Bahia, this question was given a specific social dimension in the discourses promoted through popular media or medical consultations where the *descontrolada* (uncontrolled) self was presented as posing a threat not only to the self, but also to social harmony. Many women narrated their sense of frustration at not being able to express their irritation or sadness in public, in a context where strong emotions are viewed with suspicion and substantial collective effort is invested in the maintenance of a sentiment of *alegria* (joy) in the face of adversity. Leder's model can be read as a particular theorization of the mind–body relation, which, while grounded in a specific Eurocentric, male, and biomedical epistemology, provides some interesting elements with which to reflect on Bahian women's relationships to their bodies. Although the women I interviewed often expressed that they did not really think about the internal workings of the body, they gave detailed exegeses of their bodily changes. This begs the question: Which bodily processes or organs are "present" in women's everyday experience and which recede from perception and awareness?

Wombs, Hormones, and Blood: An Ethnophysiology of Menstruation

In her classic study of reproduction, Emily Martin (2001) attends to the question of the relationship between the "self" and the body. She argues that the central image that women use in the interviews she collected is one in which the self is separate from the body. She breaks this down into a series of positions that reveal, she argues, "a fragmentation and alienation in women's general conceptions of body and self" (89). The "fragmentation" between self and body that emerges from her data ranges from the idea that the body is something the self has to adjust to or cope with, that the body needs to be controlled by the self, or that physiological processes such as menstruation are things that happen to the self rather than actions that the self does. This idea resonates widely with the interview materials I collected in Bahia and with the problem that many women raised concerning the disruption menstrual cycle changes (most notably perhaps the hormonal shifts associated with the premenstruum) are felt to have for their normal selves.

The fragmentation that Martin describes finds its origin in the metaphors used in medical practice to depict the body, which present the uterus as separate from the self or describe physiological processes as autonomic and involuntary. Yet such representations are not always evenly shared across expert and lay knowledges of the body. One indication of the kinds of discrepancies that may emerge between these is the linguistic resources available to describe menstruation, which reveal that in speech, at least, menstruation or the behavior of the uterus is not considered to be entirely autonomic. In

English, the body is referred to in the third-person neuter, whereas in Portuguese—where nouns have a gender—the body or the uterus is referred to as "he" or "she." Menstruation is spoken of in a way that grants "her" substantial agency. She can be late, come by surprise, or decide not to come when she is expected. She can be heavy, or pleasant, or predictable, and her particular qualities, such as odor, viscosity, taint, and flow, are often described using vivid terms. Linguistically this construes a rather different situation from the language of "it happens to you" that Martin (2001) reports. Although women also report the inevitability of menstruation, the verb to menstruate is commonly conjugated. In popular discourse, menstruation is thereby spoken of in active terms such as menstruei (I menstruated) or quando menstruou (when I menstruate), allowing the construction of a more active relationship to menstruating in lay parlance than in expert usages. Despite living in a heavily medicalized context, within which biomedical notions of reproduction circulate widely, the central metaphors women use to speak of menstruating reveal ideas that medical professionals strive to "demystify" (to borrow a term they often use) in clinical interactions.

Although Brazilian and U.S. health provision services are marked by similar disparities in access to health, the manner in which class processes are played out in and around medical expertise is markedly different in Salvador than in the situation Martin described. Women of all classes, I found, hold less to medical metaphors than Martin's North American informants do when narrating their cycles. Martin reports that the language of failed production and menstrual blood as waste material is prominent among North American women. Her middle-class informants associate the menstrual flow with the demise of the "egg" in the sequence of events recounted by the classical reproductive account Martin so carefully deconstructs. Martin's middle-class informants, like those I encountered in Salvador, showed some discomfort when they were not able to fully recollect the details of the process. Though their memories were often complemented by comments indicating they were not sure about what was going on "inside," she notes that "in spite of their hesitations, all of them managed to get out some version of the failed production view" (Martin 2001, 106). She concludes that middle-class women have two irreconcilable versions of menstruation. The first concerns "what [it] feels like, looks like, smells like, what the immediate experience of being a 'menstruator' is like," (107) and the second consisted in some version of the biomedical explanatory model of menstruation. She proposes that this situation is reversed among black and white working-class women, who recounted menstruation essentially by reference to the experience of bleeding (108). Martin concludes that working-class women do not summon medical metaphors of menstruation as failed production despite a clear indication of knowing these because, unlike middle-class women, they "resist" them as they "have less to gain from productive labor in the society" (110). Although I also noted substantial class differences, I would not analyze these in terms of resistance/domination to authoritative medical representations. If anything, low-income women tend to strive to perform a degree of medical competence in order not to appear as ignorant, thereby embracing rather than rejecting medical knowledge.

In the interviews that I carried out with women in Salvador, not once was the notion of failed conception put forward to speak about menstruation. The explanations Martin's informants give turn on a causal relationship between ovulation ("an egg"), its nonfertilization, and the subsequent menstrual flow. In Bahian accounts, this causal sequence was never alluded to. Few women allude to ovulation in the nevertheless elaborate narratives they give of the menstrual cycle. The few who did mention ovaries (or ovules) had encountered this organ specifically through medical practices, such as the surgical removal of an ovary in one case, the experience of in vitro fertilization (IVF) or a diagnosis of polycystic ovary syndrome in several others. The only other instance in which direct reference was made to the *ovário* (ovary) was in relation to the menopause, when the ovário was said to be *falhando* (failing). With these exceptions, however, narratives of menstruation never explicitly connected ovulation and menstruation. Ovules and ovaries were seldom evoked, whereas the útero (womb) and hormônio (sex hormones) figured very prominently in accounts about reproduction and menstruation. How can we account for this?

One interpretation might draw on the fact that the womb is more amenable to sense perception than the ovaries, whose presence—in Leder's sense—is not as directly knowable.[2] This is a general, physiological specificity of the uterus, deriving from its function and the physical sensations it procures, but one that is also significantly reinforced in Bahia. Because it is traversed by muscular contractions during orgasm, menstruation, and labor, it does not have the "foreignness" of the inner body that Leder describes. I would venture that the uterus is more "present" in Salvador than it is in the United Kingdom or in France, for example. In Bahia, this organ is given intentionality and autonomy in its popular designation as the *dona do corpo* (mistress or owner of the body). Enthusiastically narrating some of the "beliefs" that the *povão* (a derogatory term for the masses) hold, one doctor explained to me that "they" think that uterine prolapse[3] is the dona do corpo coming out of the body to look for the children that she bore into the world. On another occasion, during a divination session with a *Mãe-de-santo* (Candomblé priestess), I was asked about my general state of health in order to diagnose and remedy any pathological spiritual influence on my person. I mentioned that I often suffered from menstrual cramps, but she shrugged this off as "nothing," that is, as a simple physiological rather than a spiritual problem. She explained that this was merely the dona do corpo who was *revoltada* (angry), and she gave me a prescription for a herbal infusion of *Mãe Boa* (literally, "good mother"). "When the dona do corpo revolts herself, *fica rodando corpo* ([she] circles [around] the body)." But, she assured, "it will pass with this *chá* [herbal remedy], which will make her return to her place."

The term *dona do corpo* is, however, seldom used today among urban dwellers. Despite having a medical origin, the term *útero* bears closer associations in popular uses to the English term *womb*. The útero is still the subject of considerable elaborations, and some of the concerns that previous generations of women expressed through the idiom of dona do corpo seem to have spilled over into the contemporary—highly (bio)medicalized—practices around the útero. I was often told that during menstruation it is the útero that bleeds, and as we have seen, the útero is understood to open and close with the onset and end of menstruation. Clinical exams are commonly carried out in Brazil and include an ultrasound of the uterine cavity. Such exams are requested on a yearly basis for women who are treated in private health consultations, but they are also part of the checkups that are carried out in public health services for users of intrauterine devices (IUDs). Several women I interviewed brought out the ultrasound images of their wombs, commenting on the results they had been given. On one occasion two friends began an animated debate over the reference value for a normal uterine volume, expressed in cubic centimeters, and whether this reference value changed after pregnancy.

This is the basis for my critique of Leder, whose model implies a precultural basis to visceral sense perception, suggesting that these are given in an unmediated manner. Given that the uterus is much more amenable to sense perception than Leder suggests, it is interesting that it is absent from his analysis of bodily depth disappearance. The vivid presence of the uterus in Bahian discourse on gender and the body opens up an interesting anthropological question: What viscera are invested with meaning, and which are absent, or *dys*-appear? How does sense perception (e.g., the fact that women feel their uterus more than their liver parenchyma) blend with cultural valuation of particular organs, such as the uterus? I propose that we need a much more careful account of the different kinds of phenomenological experiences afforded and culturally relayed by different parts of the "visceral depths." In Bahia, the phenomenological presence of the uterus is not disconnected from the fact that this organ is open to the outside of the body. As I argue in the remainder of this chapter, it is already partially outside the body, and like the vagina—although one step removed—it partakes in the zone of ambiguity between "inside" and "outside."

Menstrual Lore and *Corpo Aberto*

Menstruation is commonly described in Bahia as *imundo* (filthy), *chato* (annoying), and yet as affording relief and well-being. While menarche is readily welcomed as a determining sign of womanhood and referred to as *ficar moça* (becoming a young woman), it is often recounted as a traumatic experience. The vast majority of women I encountered remembered precisely the day of their first menstruation, recalling their impressions and the reactions of those around them. Many older women recounted having had absolutely no information concerning menstruation or its existence before its onset, making menarche a fairly traumatic event.[4]

Food prescriptions are widely evoked as having been carefully observed in the past or as a thing of the *interior* (rural areas). These include a prohibition on eating lemon, pineapple, certain fish, or "strong foods" such as mango, banana, pumpkin, or cashew nut. Jussara, a community leader from the peripheral neighborhood of Arenoso, explained that lemon *prende* (coagulates) the blood, giving rise to cramps because the blood becomes *preso* (stuck), impeding the circulation of "energy." Although few urban dwellers systematically follow menstrual prescriptions, these form part of the local menstrual lore that is commonly rehearsed by people, irrespective of age or class. Traditional menstrual lore is full of ideas that might be classed as sympathetic magic. For example, I was told by my urban informants that in the interior people believed that putting a pair of scissors under the bed would cut menstrual pain or that a menstruating woman was not to go into the presence of a person bitten by a snake, because this would cause them to die from a bite from which they might otherwise recover. Stories also warn of the danger for a menstruating woman to cross a snake's path, or go into the forest menstruating, lest a snake "smell" her. Activities that are commonly proscribed during menstruation include carrying weight, playing *capoeira*,[5] or preparing certain traditional foods such as *vatapá* or *acarajé*.[6] On one occasion I went to eat acarajé on a famous street corner with a friend who complained that it was *azedo* (sour) and that the *Baiana-do-acarajé* who had served it must be menstruating. The activities that were most commonly avoided by the women I interviewed were bathing in cold water, washing one's hair, or swimming in the sea during menstruation, as these were said to invert the flow of blood upward, causing headaches or, in extreme cases, the whites of the eyes to go red. Breaking menstrual proscriptions was said to confer a number of problems: heavy bleeding, pain, *mal cheiro* (bad smell), or *ficar feia* (becoming ugly).

These ideas flow from local understandings of well-being, which concern the effects of behavior or exogenous influences on the body's balance. Such ideas are remarkably difficult to characterize because they do not neatly obey any logic of cultural categorization, but are instead actively recombined in ways that both transform and allow them to endure in new forms. These ideas blend notions about the flow and state of blood with ideas about the vulnerability of the body to weather, the emotions of others, spiritual entities, or the energy of specific places. They are shaped by notions of purity and *limpeza* (cleanliness), which blend hygienist and religious ideas and can be thought of as a marker of urban Brazilian national identity in much the same way as football, samba, and *feijoada* are.[7] The term *limpeza* brings up an interesting problem for the anthropologist because the common Brazilian-Portuguese usage collapses the two English concepts of "clean" ([to] free from dirt and impurity) and "cleanse." The *Oxford English Dictionary* tells us that the more specialized English term *clean* came to replace *cleanse*, freeing up in the term *clean* the direct association with purifying from dirt or filth.[8] What has been removed semantically by this branching out of terms is, in English, the association with moral or spiritual cleansing, such as the idea of purification from sin or guilt. This linguistic purification has not occurred in Brazilian-Portuguese, affording an extremely rich and textured set of meanings to the actions and intentions that surround acts of limpeza. In this context dirt and filth carry stronger moral evaluations. In Bahia, limpezas are regularly carried out by Christian, Spiritist, and Afro-Brazilian religious practitioners alike and are understood as acting on both the physical (cleaning) and the spiritual (cleansing) levels. Bahian ideas about cleansing mingle notions of dirt, the rapid aging of materials as a result of the humid tropical climate, and energetic notions of dirt arising from blocked energy or negative feelings such as jealousy or *mal olhar* (evil eye). Together, these produce a particularly powerful sense of dirt. *Fazer limpeza* ("doing cleansing") resolves these multiple problems either through incensing, through the annual repainting of façades, receiving a *paso* (an energy "pass"), or through the prescription of a ritual *banho de folhas* (herb bath). These actions are understood by those who practice them to have the capacity to remove mal olhar, open one's path, or dis-obstruct energy blocks.[9]

Today, the notion of limpeza continues to find new expressions in the uses people make of modern biomedical technologies, such as blood donation (see Sanabria 2009). Likewise, the idiom of *corpo aberto* (open body) is recurrent in Bahian women's accounts of menstruation. Corpo aberto and the attendant therapeutics of bodily sealing act on the transformations of a body that exists in continuity with its social, natural, and metaphysical environments. Formally, techniques to *fechar corpo* (close the body) are concerned with restoring the body's capacity as a container, thus warding off harmful exogenous influences. Although corpo aberto is a potentially dangerous bodily state—associated with possession by a spirit or the devil—it is also recognized as necessary to the correct functioning of the body, specifically the female body during menstruation or the postpartum period, when *resguardos* (periods of withdrawal or proscriptions on certain foods or activities) were, in the past, commonly observed. To have corpo aberto is to be in a state of vulnerability, a notion that cuts across physical, mental, and spiritual well-being. Menstruation is explicitly described within Afro-Brazilian traditions as a time in which women are susceptible to negative influences because they have corpo aberto. Although less overt beyond such contexts, the association between menstruation and corpo aberto is regularly drawn on by women across the class spectrum, with reference to the fact that the opening of the body is understood to happen spontaneously as the womb cyclically "opens" to release blood. In a comparative study of African American medical systems (from North America and the Caribbean), Snow (1998) reveals the recurrence of the idea that women are more vulnerable when the womb is open as well as of the general idea of a body permeable to external forces. A similar logic leads many women to consider that pregnancy is likely to occur during menstruation because this is the period during which the womb is open and able to receive semen, which is understood to fertilize the menstrual blood (see Amaral 2003; Leal 1995). Although I seldom encountered such statements during interviews, many of the questions that were raised in the numerous family planning consultations I witnessed indicated the extent to which the biomedical narratives rehearsed in these clinical contexts worked against the grain of a more mechanical logic of opening and closing. This opening of the body during menstruation is also often evoked in relation to the idea of expunging—both physically and emotionally—that menstruation is said to afford. During menstruation, the body opens to release blood, a process that is often said to bring about physical and emotional relief. Women commonly speak of emerging replenished and cleansed after a menstrual period. Menstruating enables a regular removal of substance from the body, a substance that comes to be particularly charged. Thus, while menstruation is often referred to as *a saúde da mulher* (the health of women), menstrual blood is seen as particularly *sujo* (dirty).

Limpeza provides a context for thinking about menstruation, as both a messy process to be managed (using sanitary napkins or through menstrual suppression) and an energetic *fraqueza* (weakness) or a state of emotional instability, in biomedical terms. Thus, the control and management not only of menstrual blood, but also of the attendant cyclical emotional changes (such as rage, irritation, sadness) can be thought of in continuity with broader ideas about cleanliness and purity. This issue is set against the apparently contradictory statements about menstrual blood that my interviewees made, namely the purifying, alleviating effect of menstrual bleeding and its nonetheless filthy, dirty, or repugnant quality.

Situating Dirt

Anthropologists have long attempted to account for the origin of menstrual taboos and to connect the myriad forms these take to features of social organization. At the level of cross-cultural comparison these have remained fairly inconclusive, although they have generated elaborate and detailed ethnographic accounts. Analyses of menstruation arising from small-scale societies tend to relate menstrual taboo variations to forms of social organization (e.g., kinship structures, division of labor) and their symbolic expression. The focus of such accounts is on how the representation of this experience is used discursively to signify social relations and to make statements about the kinds of effects persons have on one another. Menstruation is presented in these classical anthropological analyses as pertaining to the world of interactions and discourse, and the menstruating body is seldom addressed in a phenomenological way. With the notable exception of Martin

(2001) and Buckley and Gottlieb (1988), there are few ethnographic accounts of women's experiences of and attitudes toward their allegedly noxious blood. What would an anthropology of menstruation look like if menstruation had a predominantly positive signification in the Euro-American folk models that underlie anthropological theory? My aim is to begin without assumptions about what menstrual blood is, or—at the very least—with a recognition of the multiple meanings it can hold in any given context. To do this, I attend to the specific qualities attributed to menstrual blood and examine the relationships within which it circulates.

Mary Douglas ([1966] 2002, 1970, [1975] 1999) famously viewed bodily control as an expression of social control and approached traditional society's concerns with pollution and the modern era's concerns with hygiene as rituals whose primary function is to maintain social order and the differentiations upon which it is founded. Douglas defended the view that culturally defined attitudes toward the body reflect broader ideas about the control of social boundaries. She equated the religious symbolism of a particular group, such as one that focuses on boundaries (e.g., bodily boundaries), to the social structure of the group and distinctions between a group/nongroup, for example. In this view, societies project anxieties about the group's integrity onto the body and ritually attempt to maintain group integrity by acting on the body's limits and controlling its effusions. Dirt, she famously proposed, troubles categories: it is "matter out of place" (Douglas [1966] 2002, 36). Essentially, Douglas's approach, in evoking the breaching of boundaries, puts the emphasis on bodily or social integrity. I would like to take the problem the other way, as it were, and propose that we look at issues concerning bodily boundaries as making, rather than unmaking, the body. Despite the emphasis I give here to boundaries, I do not consider them to be either given or fixed; I propose instead to call attention, ethnographically, to the process of their making. Douglas's approach, despite its attention to the circulation of objects, concepts, and substances across boundaries, retains a view of the bounded thing as given. My critique of Douglas's model arises from my view that the body's limits cannot be known a priori and that ethnographic attention should be given to practices that bind bodies without assuming a prior state of boundedness. A bodily surface may thus be located discursively at different points, depending on the way in which the body itself is understood to hold together. That is, the body's boundary varies, depending on whether it is dressed or naked and whether the context of its nudity is, or is not, made socially appropriate through certain means (e.g., with an—albeit very small—bikini). Much can be revealed about the negotiation of bodily boundaries by tracing the way in which menstrual blood is managed in its circulation across these boundaries. Menstrual blood raises questions pertaining to the enclosures of the body, be they those of the presumed natural body (such as the skin or surface orifices) or those of the social body (such as clothes).

Managing the messiness of menstrual blood and *cuidados* (care) were recurrent topics in the conversations I had about menstruation, revealing the extent to which menstruation is understood in hygienic terms. Although I did not specifically ask about sanitary products in the interviews I conducted, the logistics of their use was brought up by women of all ages. Older women, or those of rural origin, alluded to the time before modern sanitary products were available, referring to the bulkiness of the first sanitary towels that became available, or to the logistics of using and washing cloth pads. Many narratives of first menstruation hinged on learning how to use sanitary protections or grappling with tampons (although most women I interviewed declared that they do not routinely use "internal absorbents," as they are referred to in Brazil). These accounts reveal that aunts, elder sisters, or cousins—rather than mothers—were the main source of information concerning the use of sanitary products, particularly for women of older generations. A number of scholars have called attention to the role of the so-called feminine hygiene industry in making menstruation a hygienic concern (e.g., Brumberg 1993; Kissling 2006). In early twentieth-century America, Brumberg (1993) shows, discourses surrounding first menstruation center on how girls should "fix themselves," and hygienic imperatives led to a gradual abandonment of cloth pads, considered contrary to the new norms of antiseptic cleanliness that were sweeping through modern households and defining new relationships to bodies.

Curious about how menstruation is broached in schools, I met with the counselor of one of the largest private secondary schools in Salvador to discuss how the topic is broached. Menstruation, she explained, is treated both in biology classes and in the civic education classes that she dispenses.[10] During the sex education modules, she recounts, girls often exclaim that they wished they never had to menstruate. "They say: 'God help me! I don't want to have to go through all that!'" This counselor's instruction involved teaching prescriptive hygienic behavior, blending moral imperatives with idiosyncratic notions of health. Adolescents are introduced to the developmental changes they are undergoing, in which hormones figure prominently. The young people this particular health educator teaches are instructed on the importance of being attentive to the smells their bodies produce, smells she says are linked to hormonal fluctuations. She instructs them on the importance of washing their genitals twice daily with the duchinha[11] and, for girls, of the necessity of changing their sanitary towels regularly and of waxing or trimming their pubic hair to avoid "unhygienic festering." Nevertheless, she adds that menstruation is healthy and that "it brings the greatest gift that God can give: to carry a child."

While menstrual blood is often qualified as unhygienic, its cleansing properties are simultaneously foregrounded in accounts. Lucia is twenty-three and lives with her sister in São Paulo, where she is training in hotel management. We meet in her grandmother's flat in Graça, a "noble" neighborhood in the old center of Salvador where she is spending the summer. A common acquaintance has arranged for us to meet because she uses hormonal implants to suppress her periods. Before the implant, Lucia suffered from menstrual cramps and "terrible PMT [premenstrual tension]." Although she does not embrace the idea that menstruation is "unnatural," she considers it "a drag to have to go through that whole saga every month": "During menstruation . . . I would feel a different smell coming from me, which bothered me. . . . I would feel dirty during menstruation. . . . When you're 'menstruated,' even after you've washed you feel dirty. I would be swollen in the belly, I would feel ashamed of how I was, and stay at home. . . . I wouldn't go outside when I was menstruating."

While discomfort, pain, feelings of frailness, or unpleasant smells are often alluded to, many women nevertheless spoke of the relief afforded by the flow of blood. This flow, however, needs to be carefully managed, as decades of menstrual advertisement have taught women. Thus, it is perhaps unsurprising that fear of accidents or staining are a major concern.

Janaína is twenty-nine when we meet. She grew up in a small rural community in the interior of Bahia, where sanitary products were a luxury and women often still used cloth pads. Her parents work the land and she and her five siblings lived in a one-bedroom house. Her first period came when she was only nine years old. Given that she had an elder cousin, she had some notion that something would happen to her, although it came as a shock. She recalls that menstrual blood was seen as "sujeira (dirt), that it was imundo (filth)," and that she was instructed to dissimulate her bleeding, something she found difficult in these conditions. Bleeding through one's clothes is the cause of tremendous embarrassment, and something that happened to her several times, such as during church service, which she recounted with emotion. Part of the difficulty of this event stems from the fact it was about learning *vergonha* (shame), and about being *cobrada* (called to account) at such a young age for failing to manage the effluence of blood: "I remember that my mother became extremely embarrassed when she realized that the boys had realized that I had . . . that I was bleeding. A mark had appeared on my clothes. I did not realize. And she *cobrou* [called me to account about] this. As if I should have been more careful, I had to hide it, *really*. And in the church I remember that my aunt signaled to my mother. Because I had not perceived, and my mother gave me a signal, indicating that I had to *cuidar* [care]: 'you have to look.'"

This account shows that the shame associated with the inappropriate public appearance of menstrual blood has to be taught to the young girl, revealing that it is not self-evident but the product of specific and historically situated cultural attitudes toward menstruation. As Martin (2001, 93) notes, not only must this mess be privately managed, but the mechanics of concealing it must themselves be hidden. Access to the means that enable what is considered a "proper" management of menstrual blood is unequally granted. For many of the low-income women I interviewed, the cost of sanitary products represented a substantial burden, a fact that some Brazilian advocates of the menstrual suppressive Depo-Provera injection put forward.

Managing menstrual blood presents specific challenges in domestic spaces where privacy is not always guaranteed as a result of situations of poverty or, on the contrary, to the presence of domestic employees. Accounts of staining reveal concerns with the way in which the demarcation between private and public spaces in Bahian households is managed. Maria de Jesus, an extraordinary woman who was unsure how many years beyond eighty she was and who had borne fifteen children, drew connections between menstrual and postpartum resguardos, presenting these in terms of the difficulties of effacing blood from the view of visitors.

> If you went back to work before one month had passed [after a birth], it would bleed a lot because the dona do corpo [mistress of the body/uterus] would come out, you had corpo aberto and the menstruation would come down. . . . Because we didn't have child in the maternity [unit], it was all in the hand of the midwife, so you had to lay down for four days and couldn't get up because it was normal birth and you couldn't go out because it was so much blood. [One] soiled so many clothes, my daughter!

So many. And this was a huge shame that women had, no one could look there. When a *visita* arrived, you wouldn't even hear of a man going into the woman's room! And the girls would steal a look at the baby, and the women would say: "girl, look and see if you can see a stain of my clothes."

Another woman reminisced how her mother and aunts had used washable pads when she was growing up, which itself made menstruation a less private matter. She grew up in a peripheral neighborhood of Salvador, where "everyone knew everyone's business," and the neighbors would see the pads on the wash line and comment: "*Fulana ta de boi*" [Thingy's got her period]. Many households are not equipped with washing machines, and when they are, laundry is often managed by an *empregada* (domestic worker). Perhaps for these reasons, women tend to wash their own underwear and any items that are stained with menstrual blood regardless of whether the person who habitually washes their clothes is a kinsperson or an employee. When it felt appropriate, I asked my interviewees about sex during menstruation. Most indicated that this was conceivable only with someone with whom they had great *intimidade* (intimacy), mainly because of the ensuing mess that was a cause of embarrassment. Women repeatedly expressed a concern that they would *melar* (make sticky/messy) the sheets, and when this happened they took responsibility for cleaning the sheets themselves. This labor economy around menstrual blood management and the effacement of eventual stains highlights some of the complex issues surrounding the domestic work that takes place in Bahian households. Whether women contract domestic workers (as many middle- and upper-class women do) or carry out domestic work for their own kin, they tend to take responsibility for washing their own blood.

Middle-class households often have a structural demarcation between "social" spaces, for receiving *visitas*, and "service" spaces for employees, with separate "social" and "service" entrances (on space in Brazil, see Holston 1989). Even the very smallest of middle-class Salvadorian flats have *dependencias* (domestic quarters) with a separate toilet and shower, demarcating the spaces in which employers' and employees' bodies circulate. These examples indicate that the household is not a completely private space, but one permeated by all sorts of relationships with the outside, or excessively proximate and potentially nosey neighbors, in popular neighborhoods. Containing and effacing menstrual blood and managing substance circulation in such contexts pose specific challenges. But these accounts also show that it is not the blood itself that is considered dirty, but the context of its appearance. So although it is important to consider the role of the female "hygiene industry" or of medical discourse in constructing menstruation as unhygienic, I would like to push the analysis of menstruation as a hygienic concern further by considering how the management of menstrual blood partakes in the process of demarcation between the inside and outside of bodies.

Menstrual Blood: The Inside, Out

This relation between depth and surface is particularly evident in gynecological examinations. Gynecological examinations are routine in Brazil and a key manner in which women's bodies are scrutinized by biomedicine. During gynecological examinations, and given that the focus of attention is partially concealed within the body, the emphasis on making visible and bringing into view is striking. But what happens when menstrual blood comes into view in these contexts? How is appearance of this blood, which is carefully effaced in other contexts, managed during clinical encounters? Menstruation is a central topic in family planning consultations, which often begin quite abruptly with the question: "When was your last period?" The choice of a contraceptive method is often determined by a woman's experience of menstruation: she may be deterred from using an IUD if she has heavy or painful periods, or encouraged to use a contraceptive pill if her cycle is irregular. While menstruation is discursively central in these encounters, menstrual blood at times also appears. Women who chose to use the IUD as a method of contraception are requested to come into the clinic when they are menstruating because the cervix is dilated, facilitating insertion and ensuring, for the doctor, that the patient is not pregnant.[12] On my first day in one family planning center, I was given a white lab coat and allowed to sit in on the morning consultations with Dr. Túlio and a female medical student. The first patient came in and was asked to set up in the adjacent examination room. When we entered and took place in front of the examination table, the doctor's only comment was, "you sure are bleeding a lot!"

Given the foregoing discussion, women tend to be acutely embarrassed in this situation. However, menstrual blood is seldom a cause of disgust in clinical contexts, although it is also carefully managed here. Jokes or comments are a means of circumscribing this blood. For example, later that same morning, a woman chatted animatedly throughout the consultation, apologizing about the flowing blood. She was very relaxed (something that stood out as exceptional) and did not budge when the speculum was inserted. As the doctor proceeded to clamp the cervix and measure the depth of the uterine cavity, she went on chitchatting normally. The doctor, surprised, signaled to us out of her view, with a raised eyebrow and a jolt of the head in her direction, that she had not felt a thing. Once the IUD was inserted, he removed the speculum, and the flow increased. Again, she apologized: "Desculpe, 'ta um rio" (Sorry, it's a river), but reassured the doctor that she had taken care not to stain the bed linen. When she was dressed and came out to the consultation side, the doctor joked that she should get a contract testing for sanitary product companies. All in all, however, few comments were made about menstrual blood in clinical contexts. I initially found this intriguing in light of the way in which this blood is spoken of outside the clinic.

The fact that menstrual blood, like other bodily substances, is treated with remarkable normality in clinical contexts suggests that—even where menstrual blood is culturally marked as dirty or unhygienic—disgust is not a property of the blood itself, but of the context in which it is found. Drawing on her ethnographic work in French hospitals, Pouchelle (2008) argues that mastering disgust with regard to bodily humors is part of being a good (medical) professional and that failure to do so is seen as a professional failure. Professionalism thus involves the establishment of sufficient distance to overcome disgust. In my experience, when menstrual blood formed part of the medical examination, it was normal and not a cause of disgust for doctors. One doctor did not even use gloves for IUD removals or insertions, although her dexterous use of the instruments meant her hands did not come into direct contact with the patient's body or bodily products. Similarly, during vaginal or cesarean births, blood flows freely, often onto the obstetricians' ward-clothes or shoes, with no apparent discomfort. However, once the specific protocols that produce persons as patients and patients as bodies (and their fluids and parts) have been removed, and the full social person reappears, menstrual blood is commented on in a way that signals a move from the blood legitimate within normal clinical practice to the more ambivalent blood of the person. I read this ambivalence about menstrual blood as centering on the management of the transition from both the inside to the outside of the body and from the passive patient-body to the (social) person.

These cases invite us to ask about the conditions under which disgust arises. As we have seen, Kristeva (1982)—after Douglas—proposes that excluding "filth" is the means through which the "subject" is constituted, against which it defines itself. In shifting the focus from sociology to subjectivity, Kristeva introduces a radically different notion of the boundary from that proposed by Douglas. In Kristeva's work, boundaries are ambiguous surfaces of negotiated possibilities. Boundaries divide the interior of the body from its exterior, but there is nothing given about where the boundary between the inside and the outside is. One example, from a markedly different context, is given by Strathern. She describes how the Mekeo of Papua New Guinea understand the body's topology: "The inside of a Mekeo person's body includes or encompasses an outside. The digestive tract and abdomen is not regarded as the innermost part of a person but, to the contrary, as a passage connected to the outside world, which makes it an appropriate repository of food: The tract is part of the outside that is inside the body. Conversely, wastes from the inside body accumulate in the abdomen and are regarded as the body's interior extruded so it appears on the outside" (Strathern 2004, 10).

The management of menstrual blood can be read as an effort to police this boundary between inside and outside. Kristeva and her commentators propose that female sexuality is represented as uncontainable flow, seepage, a vessel both containing and contained, and that this inherent permeability of the female body affronts the subject's self-identity, is read as danger, and as a "testimony of the fraudulence or impossibility of the 'clean' and 'proper'" (Grosz 1994, 193–94). The question of what belongs to the body, and where its delimitations lie, is deceptively clear-cut, even in contexts where the body's natural integrity is seen as relatively self-evident. Excretion and menstrual bleeding continually re-attest to the porous nature of bodily boundaries, problematizing not just the boundary between inside and outside but the very distinction between them. The vagina and the blood that flows through it are thus problematic limitrophe zones. Is the vagina inside or outside the body? The following extract from one of my field reports attests to the difficulties this question raised for me:

> The doctor spoke as if she, the patient, were completely absent. Like all patients I saw, she had shaved neatly, and the set-up of the examination table and sheet made her appear almost disembodied. As she lay waiting for the examination to begin, blood emerged from her vagina. Despite the clinical set-up, which rendered the patient's body closer to the classic textbook illustration, the red blood that seeped out attested to

something else. It was contentious in its effluence. Having commented casually on the *afastamento* (lapsing) of the vaginal muscles in terms that implied something about the patient's sexuality, Dr. T. put on some fresh plastic gloves. Without a word of warning, he introduced the metal speculum, proceeding in explanatory mode as he shone the light into the canal made by the speculum. This immediately filled up with menstrual blood, and again he commented on how much blood there was. "*Ta vendo* [See]?" he asked. This was all about seeing. Seeing inside. This rapid technical gesture, performed with the speculum, transformed the vagina. The speculum produced a separation between the inside and the outside of the body, disturbing the boundary that, notwithstanding the leaking blood, had enclosed the inside of the vagina from view. While the neatly trimmed vagina that patients present for the gynecological examination is a boundary of sorts (an object that conceals its inside), the menstruating vagina betrays the exuding attribute that social practices of managing menstrual blood attempt to conceal. (Fieldnotes: *Creating a Vista*, October 2005)

The vagina thus emerges as a kind of threshold or zone of ambiguity between the inside and the outside of the body. This explains the way in which the relative openness or closedness of the vagina is carefully negotiated throughout gynecological examinations, with doctors encouraging women to relax and open their bodies, thus facilitating the examination. Yet this situation simultaneously provides a context for substantial disquisition on vaginal tightness, revealing that laxness tends to be viewed negatively. On one occasion, after a curettage, a woman in her mid-forties lay unconscious on the examination table of a public hospital. The marks on her body gave an indication of her humble background. The doctor called my attention to the limpness of her transverse perineal muscles. Pointing to the way that the musculature had "sagged," he inserted three gloved fingers into the patient's vagina, shaking them while stating: "*Olha pra essa vagina tão frouxa, os músculos estão todo afastados, essa mulher deve ter parido um bocado de filhos*" [Look at this totally loose vagina, the muscles are all lax, this woman must have birthed a bunch of children]. This "lax" vagina seemed to index for the doctor what many middle-class Bahians see as an "unbridled" reproductive capacity among the poor. For women of all social backgrounds, being "closed" and being "open" (symbolically played out in the gynecological examination) are both valued at different moments, which accounts for the diversity of ways in which these procedures are experienced. Ideals of virginity, such as closedness or tightness, coexist with sexual imperatives of openness, as epitomized in the idiom of *dar* (to give, sexually).

One morning, among a steady flow of family planning patients, a woman of twenty-seven entered, requesting a *plástica vaginal* (postdelivery vaginoplasty) because following her two vaginal deliveries, she feels *incomodada* (discomfort). When asked what contraceptive method she uses, the woman answers that she is sterilized: "My husband likes pleasure and with all that AIDS out there . . . He likes other women, he does not respect me. I'm going to do that test. . . . Doctor, if a man has thick sperm, does that mean he is having sex with a *mulher de rua* [literally, woman of the street]?"

The doctor explains that the two things are unrelated, but that she needs to communicate with her husband and make sure they use condoms. Then—guessing her meaning—he adds: "The surgery won't protect you of the illness, you know." When she leaves, having explained that her husband refuses to use condoms, he turns to me, shrugs his shoulders and shakes his head, at a loss. This reveals how ideas about corpo aberto (open body), one's vulnerability to infections or affections of varying sorts, are managed through work on bodily boundaries and thresholds, such as the vagina.

This focus on the capacity of the vagina to be sequentially open or closed attests to the complex and ambiguous responses that the body's interiority may elicit. Zones of contact between the inside and outside are subject to careful management, as are the substances that pass from the inside, out. According to Kristeva (1982, 53), the power of the "horror within," which is constantly irrupting upon the clean and proper self, arises from the fact—within the Western context in which she grounds her analysis—that the body's inside is coded as unclean. Returning to the clinical context, we can break this down further, as not all parts of the body's interior seem to carry the same valency of uncleanliness. Pouchelle (2008), for example, notes that in French hospitals, surgical interventions on organs connected to the outside of the body (e.g., lungs, digestive organs) are referred to by medical professionals as *sales* (dirty), whereas ones on organs that are not connected to the outside of the body (e.g., the heart) are *propres* (clean). This classification originates in infectiology and serves to organize the sequencing of surgical interventions in operating theaters, whereby clean surgeries come before dirty ones. I suggest, based on the data presented here, that it is not so much the inside per se that is "unclean" but the various conduits that lead from the inside, out.

Kristeva (1982) sees, in the transition from the semiotics of biblical abomination that characterizes the Old Testament to the Gospels, the rise of a new kind of subject who has interiorized abjection. Defilement, in "Christic subjectivity" (113), originates not from the outside but from within. The internalization of defilement—which in Leviticus is given material form— and its combination with moral (symbolic) guilt produce "Sin," which in the New Testament is already inscribed in the flesh. In this process, the demoniacal–divine axis is elaborated onto the distinction between inside and outside. As Kristeva puts it: "It is the building of that archaic space [the boundary between inside and outside], the topological demarcation of the preconditions of a subjectivity, qua difference between a subject and an ab-ject in the be-spoken being itself, that takes over from earlier Levitical abominations" (117). This attests to the emergence of a form of subjectivity that is intimately connected to the production of a particular idea of the body's interiority. This visceral interiority, where ideas of the self emerge for the Christian subject, is carefully monitored, probed, and scoped by the women whom I encountered in Bahia—which is perhaps unsurprising, given the profoundly religious tenor of Brazilian social life. However, the exhortation to know oneself from the inside out, so to speak, is increasingly a medical and not a religious one.

Conclusion

This chapter has attended to the dynamic relationship between the inside and the outside of bodies as it gets played out in and around experiences of menstruation. In the first part I examined the ways in which women's experiences of menstrual cycle changes center on a disjunction between different aspects of their internal bodily processes and their ensuing sense of "self." This is often narrated through the use of the image of an irrational and uncontrollable self, erupting from the domain of the somatic out into the domain of interpersonal relations. In the second part I examined how Bahian narratives of menstruation mobilize certain elements of the classical biomedical reproductive narrative rather than others. I account for the prevalence of the womb and of blood and the absence of ovaries in these accounts in terms of Drew Leder's model of bodily *dys*-appearance. This is set against local characterizations of the womb, as a viscus that is open to the outside of the body, thus partaking in a zone of ambiguity between inside and out. My analysis of the way in which menstrual blood comes to be coded as dirty, or not, centers on the way in which it passes from the inside of the body, out. When speaking of the experience of bleeding, women often evoke the sensation of *coagulos* (blood coagulates) passing out of their body, a term that captures the viscous quality of menstrual blood and gives a sense of boundary in a way that blood *flow* does not. Coagulos don't leak; they precede outward from the body, producing a sense of inside and outside. Menstrual blood has a particular material tangibility as a substance and engages a range of social relations that are managed in a variety of different ways. I argue that the analytical focus should be on the relations that are produced around ideas of dirt and on the manner in which, within particular relationships, menstrual blood is or is not produced as dirty. I have suggested that, in Bahia, it is the place such blood occupies, its provenance—whether it is in the bin on an unconcealed sanitary napkin, in the toilet one sits on after someone else, one's own blood, a patient's blood in the clinic, or a lover's blood—that carries the potential to disgust or not. Finally, I propose that it is not so much that what emerges from the inside of the body is marked as dirty but, rather, the manner in which the effluence is managed. In this sense, it is not so much the body's interiority that is marked as dirt, but rather the conduits that lead from the inside, out.

Women's accounts of their experiences of the menstrual cycle bring to the fore questions concerning the relationship between eu (myself) and *meu corpo* (my body), as it is often summarized. A closer inspection reveals that these terms are not fixed, as the menstruating body is experienced as changeable, in turn affecting women's sense of self in complex and at times ambivalent ways. The body's capacities are often said to be modified throughout the menstrual cycle. Women worldwide associate a wide range of emotions with the different phases of the menstrual cycle (see Shuttle and Redgrove 1978; or Walker 1997). The women I encountered in Bahia at times narrated feelings of heightened insight; modifications in perception; greater feelings of vulnerability, anger, depression, or irritation; as well as increased sexual desire or feelings of renewal. What emerges from this is a sense of the cyclical, changeable body that differs from—and to some extent challenges—the normal, stable body.

Leder's model of normal embodiment, as a state in which the body is absent from awareness, is interesting in that it attempts to account for the difficulties that arise when the body is drawn out of its concealment, such as before, or during, menstruation. Although it is clearly limiting to categorize menstruation (or pregnancy, aging, and disease, for that matter) as moments of *dys*-appearance, this model is useful to account for the way in which the heightened body awareness brought about by such phenomena is commonly experienced as problematic. In juxtaposing the "dys-appearance" (the explicit awareness of the body accompanying "problematic states") and the habitual "disappearance" of the body from normal healthy embodiment, Leder attempts to account for how the dys-appearing body comes to be marked as "away" or "apart" from the self. However, much of his emphasis remains on the pathological or negative connotations of *dys*, which makes his analysis rather limited in the end. He is not concerned with questioning why menstruation, pregnancy, aging, or illness is experienced as problematic, stating this instead as fact. While this fact is certainly disputable, it nevertheless resonates with the experiences relayed to me by many of the women I met. As a model, it is useful inasmuch as it allows the formalization of the ideal (absent) body against which much of what is said about the experience of menstruation, as disrupting this normality, can be understood.[13]

This model also attempts to schematize the complex traffic between the interior and the exterior of the body, or—in Leder's terms—the visceral depths and surface perception. Menstruation, and menstrual blood, which flows from the womb and through the vagina, is interesting precisely because it reveals how surface and depth are intertwined. However, menstrual blood is largely unaccountable, for Leder, because it does not obey the logic of the visceral/surface distinction upon which he relies, and constantly threatens to surface, refusing to belong to either domain. As it flows from the purportedly absent depth, and is turned ecstatically upon the world, careful management is required to contain or efface this blood. The traffic of information between depth and surface takes on specific forms in Bahia, I have argued. Leder's model can be put to work in this context to ask about the importance of techniques that seek to bring the "visceral circuitry" to the surface and make them known. It can provide elements with which to understand what Duarte (1999) has called a fetishization of medical imagery techniques or blood tests. These, according to Leder (1990, 53), allow for greater control over what was previously involuntary: "Self-knowledge and self-command are thus achieved through technological mediation; what was depth is artificially made to surface."

Many of the women I met who had adopted hormonal methods to suppress menstruation spoke of this as a means of regaining control over their cyclical, changeable bodies. The question of control emerges regularly in discussions of menstruation. The term *descontrolada* (uncontrolled) is often used to characterize excessively emotional women or is adopted by women themselves to speak of the emotional disruptions they associate with the premenstrual period or climacteric. This means that a number of women I encountered experienced their cyclical bodies as ill-adapted to the social demands made of them. Whether it is the *fraqueza* (weakness) or reduced productivity associated with menstruating itself, or the emotional "rollercoaster" some women experience prior to menstruation, the cyclical changes brought about by the menstrual cycle are often negatively experienced, as a loss of control over the body. In this context the body's plasticity is experienced as an obstacle to everyday goals, and intervention is sought to restore the body to a balanced and fixed state, as we shall see in the following chapter.

CHAPTER 2

IS MENSTRUATION NATURAL?

CONTEMPORARY RATIONALES OF MENSTRUAL MANAGEMENT

Periodic uterine haemorrhage is one of the sacrifices which women must offer at the altar of evolution and civilization.

—Harold Beckwith Whitehouse, *Hunterian Lecture on the Physiology and Pathology of Uterine Haemorrhage*, 1914

In 2011 the *Viva Sem Menstruar* [Live without menstruating] advertising campaign was launched by the Brazilian pharmaceutical laboratory Libbs. This included a nationally broadcast television advertisement featuring the famous *Globo telenovela* star Guta Stresser theatrically musing: "To menstruate or not to menstruate? That is the question." The ad invites women to "remove the letters P, M, and T from your alphabet" by logging on to this industry-funded website, where, it is announced, the "female version of Shakespeare's famous question is answered." While the website features a series of gains menstrual suppression purportedly brings (presented as a "right" not to suffer from menstrual cramps, swelling, painful breasts, or acne), the main benefit that is showcased is the "right to not live with PMT." The homepage message gives some indication of the contents: "Everything you wanted to know about living without PMT but were too ill-humored to ask: No Menstruation. You conquered this right." This strategy of indirect marketing gives a prominent place to premenstrual tension (PMT) in the rationale for suppressing menstruation.[1]

A recent study of 1,097 Brazilian gynecologists' practicing habits found that 93 percent prescribed hormonal contraceptives to treat menstrual symptoms or for the "convenience of menstrual suppression" (Pompei et al. 2013). Another study of 2,137 physicians (partly funded by Bayer Brazil) found that 86 percent of gynecologists prescribed contraceptives specifically to suppress menstruation (Makuch et al. 2013). The most widely used methods were extended-regime oral contraceptives or the hormonal intrauterine "system" Mirena. The study found that 99 percent of gynecologists reported using hormonal contraceptives to control their own menstrual bleeding or prescribing them for their partners, the main reason being (in 89 percent of cases) to reduce the symptoms associated with premenstrual syndrome. The authors conclude that Brazilian obstetricians and gynecologists are favorably disposed toward prescribing extended-use contraceptive regimens to induce amenorrhea on patient demand. Much of the existing literature on menstrual suppression focuses on physicians' attitudes to menstrual suppression or relies solely on surveys of women's attitudes (den Tonkelaar and Oddens 1999; Estanislau et al. 2005; Snow et al. 2007). In this chapter I draw on ethnographic observations and in-depth interviews with women to examine women's rationales for experimenting with menstrual-suppressive hormonal methods. I argue that these often center on regaining control over their bodies. I analyze the ways in which popular discourses about PMT vary between women of different classes and explore the idea that PMT is a new phenomenon. This notion was commonly relayed to me by women I interviewed who had already entered the menopause and who, while recognizing their younger kin's experience, claimed that in their time "a TPM não existia" (PMT did not exist). What do people mean when they say that PMT is something new? How can it be characterized both as the product of naturally occurring hormonal changes in women's bodies and as a new social phenomenon? The chapter examines the local forms this somewhat contradictory proposition takes in relation to global menstrual suppression discourses as they circulate in international media or industry-funded scientific literature. It explores the idea that regular menstruation is a modern phenomenon and that "incessant" monthly bleeding can be bad for women's physical and emotional health. Finally, I attend to the local meanings that are associated with withheld blood through an analysis of the parallels that are drawn between menstruation and bloodletting, on one hand, and between procedures adopted to manage or arrest the flow of menstrual blood (abortion, "bringing down menstruation," hysterectomy, or hormonal menstrual suppression), on the other.

Is (Regular) Menstruation New?

The idea that regular menstruation is "new" is an old idea, as the epigraph by Whitehouse indicates. As we saw in the introduction, however, it has gained considerable public attention since the early 2000s, which saw the global promotion of pharmaceutical marketing campaigns for menstrual-suppressive contraceptives. In this chapter I focus specifically on the way menstrual suppression advocates mobilize scientific work on reproductive endocrinology to denaturalize and pathologize regular menstruation. One of the central claims put forward by advocates of hormonal menstrual suppression is that women in the contemporary period experience more menstrual cycles than ever before. Yet menstruation has always been managed. Prescriptions, social rules, taboos, myths, dietary restrictions, and child spacing strategies can all be read as forms of managing menstruation (Belaunde 2005; Buckley and Gottlieb 1988; Gregor and Tuzin 2001; Knight 1991; Reeves Sanday 1981; van de Walle and Renne 2001). In this sense, and despite claims to the contrary, there is nothing novel or "modern" about the idea of menstrual suppression; it is essentially the techniques that have changed. For this reason, I adopt the term *menstrual management* to examine the way women in Bahia modulate and experiment with their menstrual cycles, reserving the term *menstrual suppression* to refer to practices of hormonal menstrual management.

In their review of reproductive endocrinology findings—to which recent biomedical articles supporting menstrual suppression often return—McDonald et al. (1991) mobilize a series of arguments to debunk the generally accepted idea that recurrent ovulation/menstruation is normal. They suggest that "modern woman" experiences more than 450 episodes of menstruation "for physiologically futile purposes," concluding that it is misleading to view regular menstruation as "a biological evolutionary norm," given that it is "the consequence of the marked disparity between the exceptionally greater intellectual and social development of women compared with the biological evolution of humans" (373). This points to what many in this debate view as a chasm between humans' social and biological evolution. Indeed, McDonald et al. (1991, 371) come to lament the fact that "the natural history of reproduction in our species is *obscured by social overlay*" (emphasis added). They suggest that there is no known physiological advantage for what they refer to as the "extraordinary physiological expenditures of the ovarian cycle" (392) other than pregnancy, and that designing hormonal treatments in view of mimicking such physiologically "futile" oscillations are "without merit," potentially "erroneous," or factors causing "metabolic disorder, the symptoms of which are those associated with the premenstrual syndrome" (373–74).

Although it is possible that the contemporary period of declining fertility is one in which menstrual periods have become more frequent, the historical and anthropological records on the frequency of menstruation are anything but clear. Nevertheless, it is common to read in medical texts or popular media blanket statements concerning the number of periods experienced by "our ancestors" or "hunter-gatherer" women—as if these were homogenous or equivalent categories. The only ethnographic "evidence" put forward in the coverage of menstrual suppression is that presented by the biological anthropologist Beverly Strassmann, whose work with the Dogon in Mali serves as the basis on which generalizations concerning all indigenous populations are made. Interviews with Strassmann have been widely quoted in press reports on menstrual suppression, or in the Association of Reproductive Health Professionals's numerous publications in support of menstrual suppression: "It is really a myth that a lot of women have in the industrial world that we are biologically designed to menstruate on a monthly basis," Strassmann said. "Because of these differences, women today experience hormonal exposure from their own bodies at levels that are radically higher than our ancestors experienced in the evolutionary path.... It's not the bleeding that's harmful, it's the higher hormone exposure, and we don't have good mechanisms for protecting against these kinds of novel exposures," Strassmann continues. "I think the next wave of contraceptives is on the right track if they reduce hormonal exposure" (ARHP 2004b, 5).

As anthropologist Laura Jones (2011) notes in her study of menstrual suppression in the United States, expert and popular discourses around menstrual suppression have become the sites of an unlikely juxtaposition of images of womanhood: "On the one hand is a bubbly American go-getter on the fast track, and on the other is a hardy, fecund, prehistoric hunter-gatherer. The first ... twirls through her day ... calling the shots at her nine-to-five. By contrast, the prehistoric woman ... takes care of her young children while gathering food. [These] amenorrheic women emanate from the same imagination—that of the pharmaceutical clinicians and marketers of the latest generation of hormonal contraception" (127).

Strassman, presented as a specialist of "evolutionary medicine," told Gladwell (2000, 56), in an interview for the widely quoted *New Yorker* article he published on menstrual suppression, that women's bodies are not designed by evolution to handle the erratic hormonal changes to which they are now subjected.[2] This notion has a certain immediacy to it in Brazil on account of the relatively recent reduction in birth rates. One nursing auxiliary I interviewed had been using Depo-Provera for twelve years to suppress menstruation because of painful periods. During a conversation we had over coffee, after a busy morning attending patients in a health post on Salvador's periphery, she explained to me: "Woman was made to procreate, not menstruate. It is only with modernity that woman had to *sair na rua* [literally, go out into the street/leave the household] and take charge of her own life. This is what made her menstruate."

This idea was reiterated time and time again in my encounters in Salvador. The family histories of the people I met resonated with menstrual-suppressive discourse concerning the changing social roles of women and their impact on the number of periods experienced in a lifetime. For example, Teodora, who is a thirty-nine-year-old secondary-school history teacher, explained to me in an interview, "My maternal grandmother was pregnant twenty-three times. She gave birth eighteen times and twelve children lived. Infant mortality was high then. She simply never menstruated. She was pregnant or breastfeeding her entire life. Of the twelve children that lived, seven were women. Like my mother, they were *donas de casa* [housewives], they married to have children. Most of them had between four and six children. My cousins and me, we had one or two, or none. This is the demographics of our *Soteropolitano* families, Emilia."

Luzia is a twenty-seven-year-old journalist who works in the Bahian regional state's communication department and lives alone. She explained, "My grandmother had seven children and is the perfect housewife. Marvelous food, delicious person, a dream grandmother. Her thing is feeding her children. My mother is different. She reduced the number of children she had, she only had three—and I won't have any. She had her housewife phase then she went out to take care of her own life, she worked a lot, I don't know how she did it, raising us. I have no vocation to be a housewife! I don't know if I'll have the condition to have a child."

Daniela, a nurse who works in a private clinic, narrates a similar story:

In the past, there was no contraception, women had child after child. My grandmother married at fifteen. She had a child every year. When the last one was born she entered the menopause. So she practically never menstruated. When she was thirty-five, like I am now, she was already a grandmother. My mother had three then she sterilized. I will only have Pedro. I don't want another. My grandmother's generation had six or seven children. My mother's brothers and sisters had three or four and my generation has one or two. My brother has three but the last one was an accident! Now his wife sterilized. I prefer to use Depo-Provera.

These societal shifts, and their implications for the natural history of human reproduction, are routinely portrayed in the biomedical literature as having deleterious health impacts. This literature portrays the reproductive organs as being ill-designed for "incessant menstruation." Menstrual suppression advocates suggest that modern life has re-managed menstruation, making it a regular rather than an exceptional occurrence. Lock (1993) found a similar rhetoric at work in (pseudo) medical discussions of menopause, such as the widely diffused idea that women "in the past" did not live beyond menopause, a fact also presented as an artifact of modern life, leading one commentator to claim that "human females today are monkeying with evolution" (Sheehy, cited in Lock 1993, xxvii). These are accounts of the social making the biological. As such, they invert the common idiom of the social being "after nature" (Strathern 1992a) while paradoxically appealing to a real, original biology. They are predicated on the assumption that the original biological state—purportedly embedded in the physiology of the female reproductive organs, teleologically presented as constituted solely for reproduction—must be recovered through technological intervention. Menstrual suppression using uninterrupted hormonal contraception is seen as a means of returning the reproductive organs to their "original" state. The presumed "original" state, before the intervention, can be evoked only in theory, for it is not possible to imagine what human society would look like before society itself, as MacDonald et al. (1991) hope to by evoking a biological reality before "social overlay." Drawing on Engel's discussion of how the human hand is an artifact, itself "the product of labor," Lock (1993, 372) notes that anatomical changes are always "also the products of human imagination and activity." Although the arguments put forward in the menstrual suppression debate recognize this interpenetration of the social and the biological, such as in the idea that modern life affects reproductive physiology, this is done in a paradoxical manner, by attempting to purify the natural out from the social, through technological intervention.

During fieldwork, I had the opportunity to observe a number of hysteroscopies. In this procedure, the patient is under general anesthetic and a small camera is entered into the uterus through the vagina and cervix. As the camera enters, an image of the uterine cavity appears on the screen above the patient. In one of the first procedures I observed, a private practice patient was having a checkup following irregular bleeding while using hormonal implants. The procedure was performed by a young medical student under supervision. The uterine cavity appeared on the screen. "This endometrium is beautiful," the doctor announced. It was smooth and appeared a pinkish grayish color. The diagnostic was all clear: no problem. After a brief coffee in the staff room, we returned to a second patient. She was also using hormonal implants, despite the fact that she had had a tubal ligation. Her uterus was full of white filaments and matter; it looked very cloudy on the screen, and the young trainee doctor had trouble locating the entrance of the Fallopian tubes. The doctor shook his head: "This uterus is a bagunça [mess]. She has to remove it, it's just going to cause problems, I don't know why she didn't just have a hysterectomy when she 'tied' [sterilized]."

In this section I wish to situate physicians' perspectives on menstrual suppression in the context of their daily encounters with uterine and gynecological pathologies. Brazilian gynecologists seldom work only in family planning outpatient clinics. The advice they dispense in these contexts is shaped by the work they also do in operating theaters, delivering babies or treating cancers and other more serious complaints. Session 27 of the Gynecological Endocrinology congress held in Salvador in 2006 was entitled "Video-Assisted Surgery of the Uterus: Restoring an Art Object." The session's title was inspired by a letter that Viscomi, the panel organizer, had received from a patient on whom he had performed a delicate uterine surgery aimed at removing several fibroids, sparing her a hysterectomy. The patient had written: "Thank you for restoring my precious crystal. Our baby girl was born last month thanks to you." The panel aimed to question the high rates of hysterectomy practiced in Brazil, often performed on patients in whom fibroids have been diagnosed. The parallel between art conservation and restorative uterine surgery was sustained throughout the panel, and images of brush restoration in New York's Metropolitan Museum of Art were counterposed with those of innovative surgical techniques that lead to less scarring and better reproductive outcomes for patients. During the panel, films and images of the diverse uterine pathologies that gynecologists encounter in their clinical practice succeeded one another, each more horrific. A heated debate arose in the conference room concerning endometrial physiology and the pros and cons of endocrine and surgical approaches to restore the uterus to its "normal" state. The debates centered on what the uterus's normal state is and whether regular "desquamation" is physiologically necessary, or beneficial or harmful to women's health. Fibroids are often treated with progesterone hormones such as levonorgestrel-containing intrauterine devices (e.g., Mirena), oral norethisterone, or injected medroxyprogesterone acetate (e.g., Depo-Provera) — all of which limit endometrial growth. These impede the hormonal fluctuations of endogenous hormones that cyclically bring about ovulation and menstruation. The discussions that took place during the panel session explicitly framed "incessant" menstruation as a health hazard and as the cause of the gynecological disorders that these doctors encounter daily in their practices.

The language and metaphors used to describe the changes taking place in the uterus throughout the menstrual cycle are, as Martin (2001, 27–53) has shown, deeply infused with cultural assumptions. Martin shows how texts present the monthly uterine shedding through specifically charged metaphors such as "degeneration," "discharge," "death," "deterioration," and "disintegration." She contrasts this to the terminology adopted to speak of the "shedding" and "renewal" of the stomach lining, which relies on a markedly more neutral terminology. Menstrual suppression advocates, such as those making up the membership of SOBRAGE, the Brazilian Gynecological Endocrinology Society, which actively works to promote the idea in Brazil, partake in forging specific metaphors regarding menstruation. Given the widespread media presence of some of its members, these ideas work their way into the public domain, and were reiterated time and time again by health professionals and users alike. Hugo Maia Filho, CEPARH's scientific director, publishes in international journals and is a vehement promoter of highly pathological imageries of menstruation, characterizing menstruation as an inflammatory process (a term that is particularly loaded locally). Before-and-after cytological images are used to illustrate the anti-inflammatory effects of the extended-regime hormonal contraceptives promoted by the pharmaceutical laboratories that fund his research programs (and global — first class — travel). Likewise, Coutinho argues that "incessant" menstruation has exacerbating effects on the endometrial layer, causing endometriosis, pain, and unnecessary blood loss. In his book he writes, "Menstruation is responsible for aggravating an array of menstrual cycle-related disorders and is the cause of serious diseases such as premenstrual syndrome and endometriosis. . . . Freeing women of menstruation significantly reduces the risk of life-threatening disease such as ovarian and uterine (endometrial) cancers" (Coutinho 1999, 159).

Against these positions, the solitary voice of Nelson Soucasaux posits that "periodic menstrual desquamation and reconstruction" is a "fundamental feature of the endometrial physiology."[3] This unconventional gynecologist is one of the few in Brazil to publicly question and discuss the thesis of menstrual suppression. There is a remarkable absence of public opposition to these ideas in Brazil.[4] Soucasaux has a private practice in Rio de Janeiro and has published widely on "psychosomatic gynecology" or on the "archetypes of the female sexual organs." His position is to renaturalize the physiological processes associated with menstruation. In a post presenting his objections to menstrual suppression on the virtual Museum of Menstruation website, he argues that "the endometrium was designed by nature to be constantly renewed." At stake here is a debate concerning the function of the uterus and the hormonal fluctuations of the menstrual cycle beyond reproduction. This indicates the extent to which the noncyclical (male) body remains an implicit norm, for any variation thereof is seen to require assessment in terms of potential function, gained or lost. As feminist critiques have noted, sperm production in the absence of reproduction is not qualified as "unnecessary" or "wasteful," let alone pathological.

Rationales of Menstrual Suppression

One of the main reasons that the women I interviewed gave for adopting menstrual-suppressive hormonal treatments is the desire to control changes in their bodies and moods that they commonly attribute to PMT (or *tensão premenstrual*, TPM). The medical qualification of menstrual cycle–related changes in mood and well-being as a treatable dysfunction is often attributed to Frank (1931), who coined the term *premenstrual tension*. This was requalified by Greene and Dalton (1953), who considered that premenstrual symptoms included cognitive, autonomic, central nervous system, and behavioral affectations as well as mood alterations. Despite widespread popular adoption of the terms PMS or PMT and a booming literature on the topic,

PMS remains a slippery and ill-defined category.[5] Epidemiological estimates vary wildly, from 1.8 percent of women of reproductive age to 40–50 percent experiencing some symptoms, and there is little agreement on possible etiology or treatment. As Emily Martin (2001) has shown, PMS was, from the outset, given an explicitly hormonal etiology. Frank considered that it was caused by the tide of ovarian hormones that wash over women periodically, an enduring idea even today, despite evidence that there is no difference between the cycles of women who suffer from PMS-related symptoms and those who do not. Bancroft (1995, 787), a psychiatrist and former director of the Kinsey Institute, argues that the hormonal etiology of PMS is "a blind alley." While acknowledging the importance of recognizing women's experiences, Walker (1995) questions the inadequacy of current models of PMS that rely on an unproven linear relationship between ovarian function and symptom. She points to the lack of reflexivity that shapes research and much clinical practice surrounding PMS to the cultural context of symptom experience. "What does the term PMS mean to people and why is it so powerful? . . . what function does the existence of PMS (or the stereotype of PMS) have for individuals and for the society as a whole?," she asks (798). These are questions I wish to address through the analysis of Bahian women's narratives of their choices to suppress menstruation.

Ana Maria is twenty-seven years old. She works for a large publicity firm in Salvador and has been using the menstrual-suppressive intrauterine Mirena for nearly three years when we meet. She explicitly describes menstruation as a process through which she would lose control over her body: "I'm very *atenta* [aware] to my body. I eat well, if I start a cold I buy a vitamin, a fruit complex. I'm lucky because I am resistant, you know? I have a great capacity of regeneration. And with TPM and menstruation, I would feel bothered . . . because, you see, normally, I have power over my body. And that is what bothered me most with TPM, with menstruation, because I would totally lose control over my body. And that was a prejudice for me."

Aside from the feelings of weakness and the anemia brought about by menstruation, Ana Maria explains that she would feel depressed during the premenstrual period. She would become *mole* (soft/frail), without energy or *disposição* (disposition, desire), finding it difficult to get out of bed, or feel very irritated and have a lot of *nervosismo*. During PMT she would become "pessimistic" and "irrational." Hormones have an essentially negative meaning for her, and she jokes that she calls them her "enemies." When people around noticed how sad she would become, she decided it was time to take action and treat herself. "I knew that this thing [PMT] was coming from inside me and that bothered me a lot. I wanted to do something about it, but *nao tinha jeito* [there was nothing to do]. Taking a *remédio* [medicine] might improve the menstrual cramps, but it did nothing for that feeling of depression and weakness," she explains. She does not miss anything about menstruating, now that she uses Mirena. "I used to feel sick when I still had my menstruation. It's not natural. For me, it's a *doença* [sickness]," she concludes. Ana Maria's rationale for suppressing menstruation is quite typical in that it centers on bringing the body back under control. Although the emotional or physical "alterations" women associate with PMT vary widely, a common thread in such narratives is that of a body gone astray and out of one's control.

Lívia, a graduate student in the faculty of orthodontics, voices a similar idea, but places the emphasis differently. She explains that menstruating makes her aware of her body's limitations and fragility, qualifying menstruation as an inherently biological process that connects her to the cycles of nature and to the changeability of all things.

> My cycle shows me that I cannot be strong all the time. It's two things. Menstruation brings a feeling of fragility and weakness, but this is a good thing. Men have to be potency [sic], to be strong. Women pass through this monthly fragility. This is why they end up being stronger, they learn how to deal with difficulties. Menstruation brings women the opportunity to be weak.... It's a time of *recolhimento* [introspection] during which they can get in touch with their feelings. Some people experience this in a negative manner, but for me when I slow down I realize this is an opportunity to *se pensar* [think myself] and to look at my life differently.

On the emotional level, having a menstrual cycle makes her aware of how quickly everything can change, how differently things can look from one week to the next. She jokes about these radical shifts in perception, and how she tends to be more aware of shifts to a negative state of mind, such as during bouts of PMT. For Lívia, the changes brought about by her menstrual cycle are quite real, but these need not necessarily be experienced as a loss of control. For her, they offer the possibility of greater self-knowledge and are a sign that she needs to adopt a different pace. As Emily Martin (2001, 125) has noted, however, women generally "do not treat the cyclic change they experience as legitimate enough to alter the structure of work time." Many women simply do not have the possibility or control over their work and domestic arrangements to modify them in accordance with their bodily experience. Martin shows that women themselves are perceived as "malfunctioning and their hormones out of balance rather than the organization of society and work as in need of a transformation" (123). Ana Maria and Lívia experience similar changes in their bodies but interpret and deal with them very differently. These two examples reveal that the issues at stake in defining premenstrual symptoms and their appropriate recognition must attend as much to the social context in which menstrual-related symptoms are experienced as to endocrine factors per se. Reducing the myriad experiences women have of their cycles to biological (mal)function does little to explain these experiences and their variation among women and within a woman's life.

Like many women who recognize their cyclical changes through the language of PMT, Miriam, a thirty-two-year-old music magazine editor, speaks of "discovering" hers, a discovery that, in her case, was relational: "I did not have a perception of my TPM until I had a relationship with a woman. I discovered her TPM first. She would become very *descontrolada* [uncontrolled]. So it was a relationship with a woman that marked the awareness of this sensibility of mine. And as we were two cycles, the PMT was very strong [laughs]!"

When I ask her about the changes she feels during PMT, she explains that for her, the emotions vary as a function of the relationships she has with people. She always feels PMT in the context of tensions that preexist in particular relationships. With her brother, whom she lives with, she feels *raiva* (rage) and shouts about things that normally don't bother her, like leaving the toilet seat up. When she "is" TPM—as women often refer to it—this makes her furious because she feels that he has no consideration for others. In relation to her mother, TPM involves a sentiment of *culpa* (guilt). She notes that she is often embarrassed after the expression of strong emotion because—however legitimate the feelings may have been—with PMT their expression is often "excessive." This notion of emotion out of proportion is recurrent in women's narratives. While this emotion is at times characterized as "irrational," it is often felt to be underlaid by a legitimate emotion, but to be inappropriate in its form, intensity, or timing. Like many of the middle-class working women I met, Miriam works two day jobs and attends university in the evenings. Although she speaks freely about menstruation with her classmates, she never evokes her periods in professional environments. She is the only woman in her production job, and although her male colleagues are young and laid back, she earns less, often feels undervalued, and explains "there is a latent kind of *machismo* and I prefer not to raise gender-type questions in my work so as not to be treated paternalistically." In this male-dominated context, she says she would never dream of missing work because of her periods and that she never lets her emotions surface there. This, however, has repercussions on people around her, she feels, because one way or another, emotions always resurface. Likewise, Nanda works two jobs, in a publicity firm by day and teaching evenings in a private media faculty. She has used an array of methods, often taking the pill continuously of her own initiative to skip a period. She is currently experimenting with OrthoEvra, the patch, which she finds convenient, although she is hesitant to use it continuously because she has heard stories of blood clots. She leaves for work early and does not come home until after 10 p.m. In the hot Bahian climate, she finds this uncomfortable, as she cannot go home between jobs to shower and she expresses that "hygiene" is a concern. Her day job is in a small office where the toilets are unisex, and she takes particular care to dissimulate her bleeding. It is a question of privacy, she adds, for men make jokes or can be disrespectful if they know you're menstruating: "They think they can explain everything by the fact that you're menstruating." Her colleagues are "very *machista*," despite all being young, she notes.

> The modern world does not allow for cramps or TPM. Maybe I do not feel them because I do not allow myself to feel them, because if I felt [them] I wouldn't be able to work. When a woman says at work that she has to go to the doctors, it makes men nervous, they don't stop her, but it's like they think she is a strange animal. They think she is subject to her body, unable to control herself. . . . I masculinized myself because deep down I know it's going to be torture going to work with TPM. I have my days but I'm generally a stable person. Here people talk a lot about the uncontrolled woman. Woman was always seen as instable, as a being with her nerves *a flor de pele* [on the surface of her skin], like—hysterical. At work you hear a lot of commentaries, if a woman is irritated, the men say she needs sex, it's really horrible. Like: "*Thingy* is stressed, her husband isn't giving her any, it's lack of *pica* [penis]. As if pica had magic powers! [laughs].

In Nanda's account, the surfacing of the interior is intentionally deactivated given the machismo she is confronted with in her work. Martin (2001) examines the changing manner in which menstruation and PMT are treated in the medical literature over the course of the twentieth century. She shows fascinating correlations between the spates of medical studies analyzing the effect of the incidence of menstrual symptoms on women's ability to work and women's shifting positions in and out of the workforce around the two world wars. During the post–World War I depression, as women were pushed out of the workforce, many studies purported to show that menstrual symptoms rendered women unable to work. At the start of World War II, Martin shows, a rash of studies found that menstruation was not, after all, an impediment (120). The massive surge in studies of PMS in the 1970s coincide with a period in which women made a massive reentry into the paid workforce, this time unaided by a major war. Drawing on this, I suggest that one way to read the contemporary prominence of discourses of PMT in Salvador is in relation to broader questions concerning women's place in the workforce, and the changing social expectations that surround their roles as mothers, professionals, and wives. "The expectations placed on our generation, in relation to our mother's are different," Andréa commented, in an interview.

> In the past you had to be a mother before all. Working was extra. Now, financially speaking but also in terms of being valued, you have to be professional. But you are still expected to be a mother. If a woman says she doesn't want to be a mother, it's like saying you don't believe in God. Or that you're a feminist, a lesbian, or a weirdo. Women are really cobrada [called to account] if they don't realize themselves as mothers. They have to be schizophrenic: good mothers, good professionals, in good shape, with good taste and always even-humored.

I met Magda in her fourteenth-story apartment in Chame-Chame, a well-to-do neighborhood of Salvador, while she was recovering from plastic surgery. A mutual friend had introduced us because she had adopted the Mirena coil for its menstrual-suppressive effects. Magda is a university lecturer of forty-one, mother of two grown children. Her daughter's recent birthday present was a lipoescultura (liposculpting plastic surgery), and she jokes that she decided, on the spur of the moment, to have surgery with her since the surgeon offered them a discount on the second surgery. As I waited for Magda, who was receiving postoperative care, her daughter entered, speaking on her mobile phone. She weaved her way around the apartment, engrossed in her conversation, explaining that she had just been with a friend who had had um ataque de TPM (a PMT "attack") in the street and lost her temper at a shop vendor. "*Meu deus, você imagina? Nao existe ficar descontrolada assim, passei muita vergonha*" (My god, can you imagine [such a thing]? It doesn't [i.e., shouldn't] exist to be so uncontrolled. I was mortified.), concluded Magda's daughter, appalled as she disappeared out the door again. Magda finally appeared, in a satin dressing gown covering a flesh-colored elastic compression girdle, apologized for the delay, and called out to the young *empregada* who had let me in to bring us coffee. She links the emergence of her "ferocious" PMT to the appearance of fibromyalgia symptoms. This "invisible disease," as she describes it, causes terrible suffering, a suffering that is compounded by the fact that it is "self-inflicted." This leaves her feeling both powerless and guilty. With the onset of fibromyalgia, she started feeling intense PMT, and during the phases of PMT, the fibromyalgia would be stronger. She explains that she would have "fits of rage," become "furiously" impatient, *nervosa*, and descontrolada. This took on such proportions that she once had a physical fight with her partner. Eventually she, and those around her, clocked onto the cyclicity of this event. Understanding that there was a hormonal basis to her experience came as a relief: "It was good to know that it was just hormonal: that I wasn't crazy." Following her recent divorce she has become a Buddhist, and in her narrative the relation between her hormones and her self is mediated through her spiritual practice.

> For me, the question that arose was the question of the relation between the hormonal and the spiritual question. I was looking to become a better person, a more loving person, a less angry and less irritated person. And when TPM came over me I was able to do monstrous things [laughs]. So everything I learn in my meditations, on my spiritual path amounts to nothing when that period comes and those bloody hormones take over me. And talking to the Lama I discovered that for the great meditators, the hormonal cycles are changed. So you can even change hormonal levels with meditation. But, for me . . . well I'm not a great meditator, so, I don't manage that yet and I have to resort to Mirena! [Laughs.] As a Buddhist practitioner you have to learn to dominate the rage. . . . I think this is where the spiritual question arises. For us to learn how to dominate hormones. And that's the way we achieve the *upgrade* [in English] from *bicho* [animal] to human being."

In the interim, Magda, like others, opt to suppress menstruation as a kind of crutch, to manage a challenging, everyday ill health and the demands they have to meet. Despite the popularity of hormonal contraceptives in Brazil, women do worry about its long-term effects (see Gonçalves et al. 2011). However, the hormônio contained in the pill and in other hormonal contraceptives is not always seen as similar. Few women elaborated on the difference between endogenous, "naturally" occurring hormônio and synthetic hormônio such as that contained in the pharmaceuticals they consumed, often stating that they were "the same thing." Many women who use nonoral menstrual-suppressive contraceptives see no relation between these and the oral contraceptive pill. For example, Livia is twenty-three, studies management, and had been using hormonal implants for five months when we meet. She explains that she had never been able to take the pill because it gives her nausea and headaches. When I ask about the hormones in the implant, she responds: "Actually, I don't make a relation between the pill and the hormônio of the implant. For me they don't have anything in common. . . . I'm not a fan of stuff you have to inject, of taking remédio [medicines] every day and all those things that makes the uterus stop ovulating. . . . The good thing about the implant is that the blood doesn't stay trapped there, because the blood isn't made with the implant, otherwise, who knows, a myoma, a cyst or something is formed by the accumulation."

Beatriz is forty-six, owns a clothes shop in one of Salvador's shopping centers, and lives with her husband and thirteen-year-old son. She has been using hormonal implants for seven years, on her sister-in-law's recommendation, because of her PMT, which she describes as "violent" and "explosive." Menstruation was always a discomfort, and her narrative emphasizes the sensation of swelling. She notes that although her husband would see her alterada (altered) every month, he thought PMT was frescura (affectation). He was initially against her using the implant, and felt that it was "absurd" to stop menstruating:

> He simply didn't realize to what extent it [PMT] was uncontrollable. I would be completely fragilized, emotional, depressed, we would argue. After a year, he perceived the difference, because really, I'm a different person now. . . . I used to have a horrible time! I had displasia mamaria [mammary dysplasia], everything would swell. I had pain in my lower back, heavy legs, I wanted to eat sweet things all the time, and that horrible sensation of heat. Não prestava para nada [I was useless]. I run marathons, and when I started using implants, my musculature became bacana [great]. Me achei um espetáculo, tudo delineada [I felt sensational/beautiful, all delineated]. And I never stopped using [them]. . . . Não me cuido muito

[I don't care for myself a lot/excessively], I don't color my hair, my nails are not always done but I do like to look after my body. I work out, I am careful with what I eat. . . . It gives pleasure to see yourself in the mirror looking good, in shorts, in a bikini. But I'm not too vain, just sufficiently. You can't be *largada* [dis-shelved/uncared for], but *plásticas* [plastic surgeries] are an exaggeration. . . . My implants are here [shows bum]. They ran out two months ago. My doctor is travelling for carnival but I'll swap them when she's back. There must still be hormônio in there otherwise my menstruation would be back. Today when I go to public toilets and see that *nogente* [disgusting] blood in the bin [grimaces]. You really get used to not menstruating!

Some women, however, are not so enthusiastic about the effects of menstrual-suppressive hormonal regimes. Alícia is an architect and was prescribed hormonal implants by her gynecologist, who suggested they would give her "the audacity of a man," on top of their convenience. However, she soon returned to the pill in order to be able to "give a monthly pause and bleed again." During our interview she self-consciously relayed her sensation of swelling: "When I used the implant, my menstruation stopped coming down and I felt myself *inchar* [swell]. And that made me imagine that it was as if because she no longer *corava* [flowed] she remained as if accumulated there in the middle of my body [points to waistline]. I decided to remove it. I know it's probably just in my head, but I felt all *entupida* [obstructed]."

I was introduced to Pricilla, an orthodontist, because she had used hormonal implants for a number of years and had "only great things to say about them," she told me over the telephone as we scheduled our meeting. She had recently had the last capsules removed because she was entering the menopause, according to her doctor. Like Alícia, as an educated middle-class professional, she sought to distance herself from the *crendices* [beliefs] that circulate about hormônio: "The effect of the implant, for me, was that it gave me water retention, a bit of *inchaço* [swelling], and weight gain; that was inconvenient. But this thing of *ficar inchada* [becoming swollen] of that blood becoming trapped there, as the *povão* [derogatory term for the masses] says, that's just the ignorance of the povão. It's only water retention."

Now that the effect of the implant had worn off, her menstrual symptoms were back, but her menstruation was *certinha* (regular), she noted not without pride. Once "she goes away," she intends to take hormone replacement therapy, but the distinction implies that the two types of hormônio do different things in her body: the former made her swell (an accumulation of something of which there was already enough in her body), the latter will simply replace what is lacking (when her hormônio "drops" at menopause). "*Repor* [replace] in the menopause? Absolutely! Woman dries up in the menopause, she becomes *mole* [mollified]. When estrogen drops, then it's craziness. Hormônio is very important. I think that human beings are basically hormônio. We are hormônio-dependent, it's what regulates us."

Mara is a twenty-six-year-old militant in the social justice movement. She comes from a rural village in the interior of the state of Bahia, and her parents are both agricultural workers, a fact that she feels places her between "two totally different realities." She was led to reflect deeply on the way social class (for this is the term she deliberately adopts, despite being black) conditions specific relationships to the body following a botched surgical intervention. After seeking a diagnosis for abdominal pains in several public health centers, she was admitted to the emergency department when a cyst on her right ovary burst. It was removed, along with her ovary. Had the surgery been performed in a private clinic, it would have been a keyhole surgery, and they likely would have preserved her ovary. Given her profile—"young, black, from the *interior*," as she put it—they removed everything and left her with an enormous scar that runs from her pubis to her belly button. In our discussion of menstruation and its suppression, Mara drew explicit connections between the suppression of menstruation, menopause, and hysterectomy. She explained that the women in her community actively seek out hysterectomies because Brazilian doctors have long offered such solutions to what might otherwise be viewed as a problem of social organization.

> There, in my interior, the women count the years: 'it's only two years till the menopause!' because they have a horrendous relation with menstruation. Menopause, I think, is the thing they most wait for. Or removing the uterus. My mother actually celebrated the removal of her uterus! That hurt me. I was very affected. Of course, I didn't say anything, but it hurt, a lot, because what she doesn't think, for example, is that this has to do with the conditions, *né* [in it]. If she had comfort, if she could stop, for example, on the day of menstruation, if she could allow herself, say to herself "I'm not going," "don't stress me," "don't *cobre* [call me to account about] anything," etc. If she could do that it would be another relation

to her menstruation, wouldn't it? But she has to be *a mesma* [the same one] every day of the month. Including on the day that she needs a different environment. Because you should have the right to rest on that day. I don't want to call it a disease, but in terms of *incomodo* [bother], it's much worst than a cold! That's what makes me feel bad for my mother, you see. I mean, it's not removing the uterus, its not suppressing menstruation, you know!

In Mara's analysis, the conditions of hardship and poverty that characterize her community and the nature of the labor that the women she grew up with do on a daily basis make menstruation a physically sapping experience. Women are expected to be strong, dependable, even-tempered—"the same one every day of the month." This, for her, explains the particular appeal of surgical or pharmaceutical solutions, which she sees as quick-fix solutions that do nothing to address the underlying social inequalities that compound menstrual-related symptoms. While Mara's analysis is pitched in class terms, Graça, a community leader and member of the Women's Policy Bureau, gave a gendered reading of these social inequalities. Graça and I organized a focus group discussion on menstruation and menstrual suppression in the *favela* on Salvador's periphery where Graça lives. The women spoke of the unequal distribution of pain, which one woman referred to as a *sobrecarga de sofrimento* (overload of suffering). The inevitability of women's pain was relayed alongside a feminist-inspired commentary on how the *patrão de fora* ("outside" boss/employer) and the *patrão de casa* ("house" boss/husband) considered women's pain as frescura (affectation or prissiness, often associated with femininity). They joked about how men cannot stand pain, feel giddy at the sight of blood, when their wives are *de barriga* (pregnant) or when they have to receive an injection. Commenting on the hardships of being a woman in a popular neighborhood, one woman exclaimed that, if she could, she would "intern herself immediately and have her uterus out" to avoid the added pain it brought.

Like the middle-class interviewees presented in the first part of this chapter, low-income women also adopt menstrual-suppressive contraceptives to manage the demands of work and motherhood. Perhaps because their lived experiences tend to be more physically taxing, they place greater emphasis on the question of depleted strength and on the hygienic dimensions of menstrual suppression. Roselene is forty-three and works as a domestic employee in two different households in the center of Salvador. Every morning except Sundays, she departs at 5 a.m. to undertake the one hour and thirty-minute bus journey from the favela where she has built her house with her own resources after two divorces. She has carried eight children, but only five lived. Three of her daughters live with her in her two-bedroom house, two with their partners and four of her grandchildren. In the households where she works, she cleans, irons, washes, and cooks food for the entire week, as well as doing the shopping, on foot. She also washes laundry for people in her employer's neighborhood and carries heavy loads of washing to and from her house on the long bus journeys. When she tells me about her menstruation, she explains that it has always been *saudavel* (healthy). She has cramping "like everyone" and lack of *animo* (energy) but she is strong and has always faced the *luta* (struggle) that is her life with resolution. She recently heeded her daughter's suggestion to try Depo-Provera because she was feeling fatigue and during her periods would get dizzy in the crowded and overheated buses. Summer, with its many festivals and carnival, were just around the corner, and she wanted to try "*essa coisa de ficar sem menstruar, curtir minha praia, usar branco todo dia*" (this thing of not menstruating, enjoy my beach, use white [clothing] every day). She explains that her periods "*parou de descer, como quando ficava de barriga*" (stopped descending, just like when I was "of belly"). However, this soon brought about a feeling of *incomodo* (discomfort) and *inchaço* (swelling). She started to feel giddy, nauseous. "This blood has to come out, when it is trapped, you swell and *passa mal* (become giddy). I didn't like to suppress my menstruation, I think menstruation is the health of women, even if it is dirty and an incomodo, even when it depletes you, that blood has to come out."

Dra Janaina works in one of Salvador's public teaching hospitals in the mornings and spends afternoons in her private practice. As such, she had much to say about the distribution of menstrual-related complaints across class differences. She explains that many of the patients she sees in her private practice consult for PMT. Each patient has "her own particular kind of PMT." While some feel anger, irritation, and headaches, others experience depression, swollen breasts, and hypersensitivity. In her words, the patients to whom she attends in the public service also suffer from PMT but just don't realize it: "More simple people think it's normal to feel this, they think it's normal to suffer and to go through these difficulties. TPM does not bring them to the doctor. To the contrary, people who are more culturally advanced complain more because they have access to a better medical service and know that it is not normal to suffer from this."

My data tend to support the fact that low-income women don't recognize their symptoms as TPM, although my interpretation differs. Suffering, for many women, is a sign of *força*, which Scheper-Hughes (1992, 188) defines as a "constellation of strength, grace, beauty and power." I suggest this partly accounts for why many of the women living in conditions of hardship whom I asked about TPM relayed the idea that it was frescura. According to Scheper-Hughes's analysis, "the rich and males" have força, whereas "the poor and females" have *fraqueza* (weakness), but it seems to me that when women spoke of TPM as frescura, they were directly challenging the categorization Scheper-Hughes relays and rejecting the equation between women and fraqueza. For example, Lucidete, a seamstress in her early thirties, is raising three children alone. We meet in CEPARH and she is keen to show that she is a responsible citizen, unlike her sister, who has stayed in the interior with their mother and her eight children. Her husband "doesn't want her to *evitar* (avoid [pregnancy]) or *estrangular* (strangle [sterilize])." She herself uses the pill continuously because she "cannot get used to menstruating." She tells me about the pains, and the lack of *animo* (energy) that menstruation would bring, and I ask her if she has ever felt TPM. "Never," she replies, firmly. I ask if she knows anyone who does and she firmly shakes her head. Given the long discussion of menstrual symptoms that preceded and drawing on the repertoire that is common in middle-class contexts, I continue, "this thing of being *nervosa*," to which she replied: "*Olhe* [look] this, for me, is frescura, *viu*? [OK?]," cutting the discussion short. On another occasion, I was preparing food for a community event with a group of women in a popular neighborhood. One woman started speaking (unsolicited, quite to my delight!) about a neighbor who has so much pain during her period that she has to go to hospital to have "*buscopan na veia*" (painkiller on a drip). Another girl shrugged this off: "That's just *mima* [being spoiled]. That's just psychological!" she replied. "When I feel pain, I never speak about it. I don't like to *incomodar* [bother] [others]." I found that low-income women—who, in the literature, are those who suffer from *nervoso*—did not identify with this diagnosis in relation to menstruation. By contrast, middle-class women, as I have shown, frequently referred to nervoso in relation to menstrual cycle changes. However, their use of the term differs substantially from that outlined in the literature on nervoso in Latin America (e.g., Duarte 1986; Rebhun 1993; Scheper-Hughes 1992), which describes nervoso within the frame of social suffering. Duarte (1986) proposes that nervoso is an affliction of the working classes, for whom personhood is nonindividualized, and illness is explained by reference to interpersonal relations. By contrast, the middle classes, according to Duarte, search for the causes of illness *within* the individual. As we have seen, however, illness emerging within the self, as is the case with PMT and hormonal changes, rather than through an external (e.g., infectious) agent, is a source of specific suffering. The fact that mood swings or physical symptoms can be attributed to hormonal fluctuations (and despite the fact that the biomedical literature contends this correlation, as I pointed out at the outset) is experienced as a relief: It objectifies the source of suffering, rendering it partly outside or "other" to the self.

To sum up, menstrual suppression is often adopted as a means of regaining control over menstrual cycle changes, enabling women to adapt to the requirements of their busy working lives, where these are experienced as depleting or challenging. A paradox emerges, however, as withholding menstrual blood is often understood to be deleterious to health, leading many women to abandon the practice. This understanding stems from the idea that regular bleeding is integral to the maintenance of health and from concerns regarding the resulting accumulation of blood in the body. In the following section I explore parallels that are made between the circulation of blood and the flow of menstruation. This reveals a humoral understanding of the body in which ideas about the management of both menstrual and arterial blood flow continue to play a central role. I therefore briefly trace how the biomedical concept of sex hormones has itself been absorbed into these specific ideas of blood.

Menstrual Management: Withholding Blood and "Making Menstruation Come Down"

The relation between the flow of arterial and menstrual blood is explicitly drawn upon by Coutinho (1999, 2007) in his anachronistic reading of the history of bloodletting. He argues that therapeutic bloodletting found its rationale in the observation that Hippocrates made of the health benefits women drew from menstruating regularly. This leads him to predict the following: just as the history of medicine has witnessed the abandonment of this practice, so too will it witness the relinquishment of incessant menstruation which, he predicts, will one day also come to be perceived as "barbaric." As we saw in the previous chapter, the widespread consensus in Bahia around the idea that menstrual blood is *ruim* (bad) stems from the cleansing function attributed to menstruation, which brings what is bad out of the body, producing waste that must be carefully managed precisely because it is charged. The ambiguity of menstrual suppression rests on the fact that while it resolves the management of "that" blood, it is seen to have deleterious effects, precisely because impurities are not evacuated but accumulate inside the body. Hormônio is understood to impede the formation of (menstrual) blood, but fears concerning how the accumulation of hormônio may lead to the formation of fibroids, cysts, or other pathological growths regularly emerge.

In this final section I place the practice of hormonal menstrual suppression in relation to the other practices of menstrual management, or menstrual regulation, in which the women I encountered engage. I do so because there is much to gain by considering the practices of regulating, withholding, or inducing bleeding together, a fact that is seldom recognized. Existent work on menstrual suppression tends to analyze this practice in relation to contraception, to the pseudo-feminist claims made by menstrual suppression advocates, or to focus on the mobilization of ideas of nature and artifice in this debate (see Jones 2011; Kissling 2013; Mamo and Fosket 2009; Manica 2011). However, my inquiry into this practice in Bahia led me to a range of apparently disconnected practices, concerned with the regulation of blood more generally, that help to explain both how and why women may experiment with suppressing their periods. In this sense I am concerned with revealing the way menstrual management rationales span beyond menstruation per se.

The distinction between contraception, abortion, and the promotion of reproductive health through the stimulation of the menses—referred to in Brazil as *fazer a menstruação descer* (bringing down menstruation)—is tenuous and has a recent history even in biomedicine (see Gerber 2002 or van de Walle and Renne 2001). Several of the women I interviewed who used hormonal contraceptives to suspend menstruation explained that there are several ways to stop menstruating: becoming pregnant, taking *remedio* (medicines), or having a hysterectomy. This creates an interesting and somewhat paradoxical relation between pregnancy and hormonal menstrual suppression, for although menstrual suppression grew out of the search for new contraceptive techniques, the relation is sustained through the idea of arresting the flow of menstrual blood. In this sense, hormonal menstrual suppression is an odd contraceptive, which, I suggest, accounts for the fact that it was often taken up as a specific project (to suppress menstruation), at times independent of its contraceptive function.[6]

Menstrual suppression and hysterectomy often were explained to me alongside each other, revealing that they are often understood along similar lines: as removing something that no longer serves a purpose. In the course of fieldwork in clinical settings I witnessed many discussions of hysterectomy and its possible benefits. The particular doctors I worked alongside tended to discourage women who sought hysterectomies of their own accord. These were surprisingly numerous, as the following exchange between a doctor and her patient revealed. It was mid-morning in a family planning clinic, and the patient, aged twenty-three and mother to three children, was weighing her contraceptive options. She was tired of taking pills and had disliked Depo-Provera, the trimonthly hormonal injection. She wanted to be sterilized. There was no way she was bringing another child into the world!, she exclaimed. The doctor abruptly explained that she did not have the right demographics: too young, not enough children to justify such a definitive solution. The woman insisted, explaining her circumstances: having to find someone to look after her children each time she came to the clinic on the long bus journey to collect methods that were not always available, forgetting to take her pills, the *meninos* (boys) who did not like using condoms. . . . The doctor sighed and began explaining that tubal ligations were counterindicated for young women under the age of 30; they commonly lead to abnormal uterine swelling, requiring full hysterectomy within five years. Lightening up, the patient responded: "God, that would be a blessing. Why don't you just remove the lot in one go, *né*?" In *The Naked Man*, Lévi-Strauss (1981, 175) refers to the distinction made in Amerindian myth between that which is separable from the body and that which is inseparable. While eyes stand for that which cannot be removed without injury, excrement is destined to be removed at regular intervals. Teeth occupy an intermediary position, as aging may separate a person from their teeth, which had nevertheless felt to belong as much to the body as the eyes. I want to use this apparently simple distinction (separable from the body/inseparable from the body) to think about menstruation. While menstrual blood occupies a position similar to excreta in this typology — in that it is removed at regular intervals — menstruating is constructed simultaneously as inherent to female bodies and as removable from them. Unlike excretion, which is a function that characterizes bodies throughout their existence, menstruation is a bodily function that starts and stops at significant moments in a woman's life (menarche, pregnancy, stress, the influence of other women's cycles, menopause, and so on). As we have seen, contemporary discussions surrounding menstrual suppression tend to center on whether, given these more or less regular intermissions in menstrual periods, menstruation is a fundamental aspect of what female bodies *are*. The task at hand is to consider this in a context where it is commonly stated that the uterus is "disposable" for women who have already had children, and in which surgical intervention routinely removes organs. There is, therefore, nothing self-evident about Lévi-Strauss's distinction in the context I describe, which invites us to consider how decisions are made about what is removable or transformable in bodies.

The medicalization of reproduction has rendered the notion of menstrual management fairly alien to most women who live under biomedical regimes. Most women in Europe (the implicit frame of comparison for this work) actually do not know that the bleeding episodes they experience on the pill are not menstrual periods. By contrast, in Brazil, where the arguments of menstrual suppression advocates have received widespread attention, this fact is comparatively well established, even among uneducated women. Menstrual suppression advocates argue that it is modern life (and its accompanying demographic changes) or biomedical regimes (such as the 21/7 oral contraceptive pill regime) that have produced regular menstruation as a norm. Ironically, it is through a conjunction of regulatory mechanisms and legal frameworks surrounding pharmaceutical packaging and prescription that biomedical practices now return to the age-old possibility of menstrual management—with notable differences in rationale, emphasis, and technique.

Emmenagogues are herbal or pharmaceutical substances that bring about the menses and are used to remedy a delayed menstrual period. Browner (1985) gives an account of how urban women in Cali (Colombia) use such substances to regulate menstruation. Emmenagogues can both remedy a delay—considered harmful because undischarged blood can lead to illness—and provide an early pregnancy test (*prueba*), for when menstruation fails to "come down" women are given a tangible proof of pregnancy. In Bahia, and in the context of the illegality of abortion, reference is often made to the "ambiguous" intentions of women who use emmenagogues. This is compounded by the ambiguity of the term *aborto* (abortion). *Aborto* is the generic term for both miscarriage and (intentional) abortion, which is illegal, in Brazil. The term is thus qualified as either *natural* (spontaneous) or *provocado* (induced). Marizete, whom I met at CEPARH, where she had come to have her hormonal implants removed after gaining sixteen kilograms, narrated her three abortions to me during an extensive interview. She is a resourceful woman of twenty-seven who lives in a small favela in the center of Salvador. Unlike most of her peers and kin, she has completed a secondary school education and has a telemarketing job, which pays for private health insurance. Jokingly commenting on the prolific fertility of her mother, aunts, and sisters, she states that ignorance and short-sightedness cause her girlfriends to opt for pregnancy in an attempt to gain autonomy, which ultimately makes them more dependent since their relationships are often short-lived and they return home to their mothers, who provide for their babies in the absence of fathers. Marizete likes the implant for its reliability as a contraceptive method and for the convenience of being free of menstruation, but she clearly associates her weight gain with the accumulation of hormônio in her body. In one of our conversations, she told me about her three abortos, referring to them as such and not as "bringing down menstruation," as other women commonly do. Her narrative distinguishes between "degrees" of abortion, evaluated on the basis of what is aborted. She carried out her first abortion alone in her mother's house, using a combination of the pharmaceutical drug Cytotec[7] and a bitter herbal infusion, as indicated by a friend's mother. In her case, she notes, only blood came out: "It was impressive, it started immediately, I had lots of pain, bled so much and had cramps." She notes that in her different experiences of aborto: "it never came to be a fetus [nunca chego a ser feto], only blood came. . . . Many women wait, in doubt, because of fear, because of their financial situation. They wait to see, but I say: 'who waits to see, sees too much.'"

Aborting a fetus is different, a point that she powerfully made by narrating the story of a friend whom she had recently helped. Calmly recounting the event, she explained that her friend had waited and that when the abortus came down, "the bag had not torn and it came out all formadinho [formed], with little hands and black hair." As we pondered this poignant image with emotion, she noted, "aí é outra coisa [this is a different thing], I will never forget that." The distinction she makes resonates with the analysis of abortion proposed by the Brazilian anthropologists Leal and Lewgoy (1995). They argue that the dichotomy between the widespread antiabortion ideology in Brazil and the pervasiveness of the practice stems from the fact that unless the physical alterations of the body that signal pregnancy are recognized, interpreted, and socially assumed as a pregnancy, then action taken to "dis-obstruct" the body by inducing blood flow is not interpreted as abortion. That is, the pregnancy is not interpreted as having generated a "person," and action taken to "bring down menstruation" does not carry the same moral and emotional implications (68–69). This analysis tallies with and enriches other discussions of the proximity of contraception, menstrual regulation, and abortion in Latin America. The common assumption underlying the demographic, family planning, and indeed Brazilian biomedical interpretation of women's "ill-disguised intentionality" in their use of emmenagogues to "bring down menstruation" is problematic in that in focusing on the cultural processes through which personhood is—or is not—attributed to the early conceptus, it runs the risk of overlooking the institutional and structural factors that produce such "cultural" differences.[8] Abortion raises numerous questions that are beyond the scope of this work, but I present this material to make two specific points regarding menstrual management (for detailed discussions of abortion in Brazil, see Alves et al. 2014; Aquino et al. 2014; Aquino et al. 2012; Guedes 2000; Menezes and Aquino 2009; Menezes, Aquino and Oliveira da Silva 2006). The first concerns the different techniques available to different groups of women, and the second concerns the ways in which these in turn affect and reenforce different experiences and understandings of the body. Abortion is illegal in Brazil (with the exception of cases of rape or danger to the mother, although there are issues of access to public services in these cases) but is readily available in private clinics to women who can pay.[9] In these contexts, abortions are carried out in safe, clinical environments that are relatively free of moral reprimand, according to the women with whom I spoke. They are carried out by suction, under full anesthetic, such that the women do not engage directly with the aborted materials. In these clinical contexts, as in contemporary U.S. and European contexts, the biomedical technologies of abortion have made the idea of "bringing down menstruation" appear as false consciousness. This has much to do with the ways in which the complex nexus surrounding abortion technologies (legal frameworks, conceptualizations of the embryo, biomedical protocols, and so on) has produced the biomedical category "abortion" as something radically different from menstrual management. By contrast, women for whom the cost of private abortion is prohibitive—such as Marizete and her friend—rely on a range of alternative techniques to induce abortion themselves. Depending on the emmenagogue taken, menstruation will "come down," or, if complications ensue— as they often do—a woman will present herself to a public maternity stating that she is having a (spontaneous) aborto.[10] Among the substances used to bring down menstruation, the most common is Cytotec. Cytotec tablets are usually crushed, combined with a cream, and applied directly in the vagina, often in combination with a "bitter" *chá de folhas* (herbal infusion) ingested orally to promote cramping.[11] I was also told of women applying hormonal injections, or mixing oral contraceptive pills in various concentrations with diverse *chás*.[12] My point is that for middle-class women who obtain clinical abortions in private clinics, techniques and procedures remove them from a more immediate experience of abortion, whereas for the women who "bring down menstruation" or provoke abortions with various substances, this experience is more direct, at times more (physically) painful, and more likely to end in death. These differences in menstrual regulation/abortive techniques and the ways in which they mediate a more or less immediate experience with the dis-obstructed blood cannot be overstated. I return to this in my discussion of how medical practices reinforce class difference in the following chapters, but I introduce this example at length here because it evokes particularly well the ways in which different techniques of menstrual management (if one sees in abortion a form of menstrual management) mediate markedly different experiences and understandings of bodies. In referring here to techniques, I mean both the conjunction of objects, *materia medica*, and knowledge practices within which these are deployed. In this respect, pharmaceutical products (e.g., Cytotec or hormonal injections) used in nonprescribed ways to make menstruation come down are not the same thing as pharmaceuticals used in approved or prescribed ways. My point here is that these overlaps (or "ambiguities of intention") are as much the product of (modern) national regulations and legal frameworks surrounding menstrual regulation techniques as they are of "tradition," as it is commonly claimed (both by doctors locally and in many social science accounts).

Menstrual Suppression and Religion

Beyond indexing health, the management of menstrual blood is an issue that is heavily invested with religious meaning. Despite the fact that most world religions place restrictions on menstruating women, I had not assumed that the practice of menstrual suppression would find support among religious practitioners.[13] Although such an analysis is beyond the scope of this analysis, it is interesting to note the way menstrual suppression has been, in places, taken up for specifically religious goals. For example, in India, there are reports of women using hormones bought over the counter under the names of "purity pill" or *pali lambaonyachi goli* (menstruation-delaying pill), particularly during the months of ritual festivities. A news article on the subject cites a doctor who notes that "even educated women" are taking it upon themselves, often under familial pressure, to use these pills and ensure their participation through labor in the ritual proceedings and to avoid the inauspiciousness of menstrual impurity during festivities (Pallavi 2005).[14] Similarly, Hartmann (1995, 192) reports a consultation process between the national Indonesian family planning board, members of International Planned Parenthood Federation, and *ulama* (Muslim religious leaders) concerning the use of extended-regime oral contraceptives, dubbed locally as "the Ramadhan Pill," to enable women to maximize graces obtained during Ramadhan without having to pay back days of fasting missed as a result of menstruation. Likewise, the Jewish Women's Health Guide for Medical Professionals advises "A woman is required to follow the rules of *niddah* when she experiences uterine bleeding. . . . However, she is not obligated to become *niddah* on a monthly basis. In fact, regular monthly menstruation is a relatively recent phenomenon. The average woman at the time of the Talmud would have menstruated 160 times in her life, compared to an average of 450 today. . . . If there is no medical contraindication, using artificial means to adjust the menstrual cycle to prevent being *niddah* is halachically permissible" (Zimmerman 2012).

The data we have in the ethnographic record on withholding menstrual blood are highly disparate, making comparison impossible. At best, the partial connections (Strathern 1991) between practices and social interpretations of withholding blood are productive through the gaps they expose.[15] In the final section I turn to some of the ways in which menstruation and its suppression are approached within *Candomblé*. Whether or not they actively partake in Candomblé religious practices, most Bahians know who their *Orixá* (deity) is and have been to a *terreiro* (temple) for a celebration. During my fieldwork, I met regularly with Dona Zuzu, a Candomblé initiate who offered to tell me about menstruation in her "African culture," as she referred to it. During menstruation, she explained, a woman has *corpo aberto* (open body) and cannot do anything involving the spirits, as when she menstruates, a woman is open to *tudo que é ruim* (all that is bad). That is, if something negative happens when the Orixás are summoned, the bad energy will *pegar* (stick) on her. Responding from her own experience, she explained that for someone who actively participates in Candomblé, menstruation is problematic, especially when the person is "of" an Orixá for whom menstrual blood is taboo, as is her case:

I am of Obatala and my menstruation went away very early, for medical reasons. I was lucky, because chance had it that at the age of thirty years I had a full hysterectomy.[16] This was lucky for me because I am initiated in Obatala and I cannot see blood at all, under any circumstances, or I become giddy and faint. That is why I am in favor of the injection to suspend menstruation. Other people are afraid of it because they think that this is the period in which women *bota para fora* [throw out] all that is negative in their body and they don't take the injection because they see menstruation as a cleansing.

Throughout our many discussions, Dona Zuzu narrated other cases of friends and acquaintances who had entered the menopause early, had opted for hysterectomies, or had used hormonal contraceptives to suspend their menstrual blood, in view of carrying out their ritual duties.[17] Indeed, a woman who bleeds is not only impeded in her ritual duties, but her power is affected, and she must dispose of her blood extremely carefully lest someone use it against her. The Cuban sociologist Ileana Hodge does comparative work on Yoruba religions in the New World and notes that in Santaria (the Cuban form), menstrual blood is not as polluting as it is in Candomblé, and certainly is not as much of an impediment to ritual practice. In the Cuban context it is men, not women, who tend to play dominant ritual roles. In her analysis, the negative power of menstruation is more contended and disputed there than it is in Bahia, where there is a general consensus that menstrual blood is *ruim* (bad). The differences are, in her view, essentially historical and political, arising out of the different contexts within which Yoruba religions developed in Cuba and Brazil, and the way this has shaped the trajectories of religious leaders. She suggests that if Bahian *mães-de-santo* (Candomblé priestesses) opt for full hysterectomies when confronted by gynecological problems, this may be linked to the way they envisage their religious careers, in a context where being free of menstruation removes all impediments to ritual practice and to taking on the succession of a temple (Hodge, personal communication). So it is not that they have a hysterectomy solely for religious motives, but that, when confronted with the decision of whether to undergo hysterectomy for medical reasons—a choice with which Bahian women are commonly faced—religious questions weigh heavily.

Conclusion

Faircloth (2013, 129) outlines the "fantasies of the natural" at work in the references made to an imagined human evolutionary past that are used to legitimize reproductive patterns and behaviors modeled on selected features of primitive or ancestral modes of being. Drawing on her research with women in London and Paris who breastfeed their children for extended periods of time as part of a "hominid blueprint" of optimal care, Faircloth argues that full-term breastfeeding rests on the assumption that humans have the same bodies as they did hundreds of thousands of years ago. This suggests, she shows, that under contemporary circumstances, our biology is understood to have become maladapted. This fetishism of the "primitive" is founded on a powerful notion, she argues: the idea that a phenomenon (like mothering practices) is really an evolutionary adaptation rather than a cultural construction of an adaptation, that is, rather than a natureculture hybrid, as Haraway would put it. This constructs culture as external to nature and "presents a dichotomy in which human interaction with, and manipulation of, the environment is considered artificial" (Faircloth 2013, 130). Such fantasies of the natural have also been referred to as "paleofantasies." In her popular science book *Paleofantasy: What Evolution Really Tells Us about Sex, Diet and How We Live*, Zuk (2013, 57) argues "The notion of a mismatch between modern and ancestral humans can be seen everywhere from diet books detailing how cavemen ate to conjectures about why powerful male celebrities seek out young women . . . we often look to our evolutionary past to explain the woes of our apparently ill-adapted present."

The proposal to suppress menstruation in order to return to ancestral patterns of fewer menstrual episodes is a typical paleofantasy, or what Jones (2011), in her analysis of menstrual suppression discourse in the United States, calls "paleo-rhetoric." The menstrual suppression paleofantasy posits that menstruation is not "natural" and as such constructs regular menstruation as a natureculture hybrid. Further, it makes a specific—evolutionary—claim about the plasticity of human bodies. The evolutionary view appealed to here is one in which bodies evolve in response to their social and natural environments. Human bodies are presented as inherently plastic or changeable in the *longue durée*, over historical time. However, debates about the end points of human evolution and the relative adaptation of human bodies to their contemporary environment (as if this were homogenous) discursively construct "our" contemporary bodies as maladaptive. There is, it is suggested, a time lag between the hard-wiring of our bodies and the rapid societal advances that render this hard-wiring (or "hormonal-wiring") pathological. The proposal to use hormonal contraceptives to suppress menstrual bleeding construes bodies as plastic in a further sense: Hormonal intervention is mobilized as a means to mold the body back to a purportedly original state. As we have seen, menstrual suppression debates suggest that biology is shaped by social life. Changing patterns of fertility associated with the entrance of women into the workforce are described by menstrual suppression advocates as exposing "contemporary" women to "incessant" menstrual periods, an evolutionary aberration that is presented as potentially hazardous. These debates around the purported misfit between our modern bodies and the inherited hard-wiring we carry point first and foremost to conceptual difficulties in how we collectively understand the historicity of our bodies. Despite the radical reconfiguration of the biological as technology and as an icon of seemingly endless cultural innovation, biology, as Franklin (2013) has shown, continues to stand for that which is fixed, given, and stable. The concept of plasticity, which I borrow from Malabou, with its dual aspect of receiving and transforming form, speaks precisely to this problem. With regard to neurobiology, Malabou (2011, 49) argues that the brain's plasticity "constitutes a margin of possible improvisation on genetic necessity. Today we no longer have just chance or necessity. There is chance, necessity and plasticity—which is precisely neither chance nor necessity" (my translation).

This chapter examined the idea that women should be able to choose if and when to menstruate in light of the reasons they give for their choice. I show that the practice appeals to an ideal of modernity, emblematized by a move out of nature made possible through technological intervention. Menstrual suppression is adopted as a means of control and monthly menstrual cycle changes as impractical, given the requirements of modern life. A paradox emerges, however, as withholding menstrual blood is often understood to be deleterious to health, leading women to abandon the practice. This understanding stems from the idea that regular bleeding is integral to the maintenance of health and from concerns regarding the resulting accumulation of blood in the body. The hormonal practices traced here show that the boundaries between the contraceptive and off-label properties of this class of drugs are blurred and, with it, the boundaries between the logics of fertility reduction, sexual control, well-being, and self-enhancement. Rather than presenting hormonal menstrual suppression as an entirely novel phenomenon, this chapter seeks to set the practice alongside strategies of menstrual management that have long been available to women. Historical and cross-cultural work on the substances used by women to manage their menstrual cycles, or "bring down menstruation," reveal the porosity of the boundaries between contraception, abortion, and menstrual regulation. The chapter therefore approaches the issue through an analysis of the *materia medica* of menstrual management. In the subsequent chapters I turn to the relations between hormonal menstrual-suppressive drugs and the bodies they transform through an analysis of their mutually transformed materialities.

CHAPTER 3

SEXING HORMONES

Hormones have become central to contemporary understandings of sex. In this chapter, I show that they are interesting precisely because they sit at the boundary between "sex" and "gender." Building on historical work on the development of endocrinology (Fausto-Sterling 2000; Oudshoorn 1994; Rohden 2008) and on ethnographic research carried out in medical congresses and among diverse hormone users, I show how sexual dimorphism has been reinscribed within endocrine practices. I begin with two mutually illuminating cases that speak for the many other instances in which hormones are made to perform gendered tasks. Testosterone is increasingly being prescribed to women, a use that is legitimated as Brazilian doctors discuss the clinical applications of androgens in gynecology, while so-called female hormones are only available to transsexuals and travestis[1] through informal means in Bahia, and information on appropriate regimens remains unavailable. Together, these two ethnographic moments illustrate the constraints that are set out by the social context in which sex hormones come to be used. They also reveal that although some aspects of sex, which can be synthesized and manufactured into drugs, can now circulate outside bodies, specific norms and prescription regimens continue to reinscribe their uses within a dualistic model of sex.

The chapter considers the way hormones often continue — in popular and medical discourse—to be sexed within a binary frame and explores a range of practices that begin to bring such binaries into question. Historian Nelly Oudshoorn shows that hormones need not have been framed within such a binary model of sex. She argues that the chemical model of sex brought about by early twentieth-century developments in endocrinology might have led to a break with the anatomical model of sex that associated sexual identity with particular organs (Oudshoorn 1994, 145). The formulation of research questions and activities was shaped by scientists' assumptions concerning the essence of sex, as located in an organ, a gland, or a chemical substance. The chemical model of sex that was uncovered implied a radical break with previous understandings, in that sex, as a chemical agent, was understood to circulate throughout the entire body. Oudshoorn describes the wonderful puzzlement of early sex hormone researchers when they gradually realized not only that male hormones occur in female bodies and female hormones in male bodies, but that estrogens were necessary in emblematically male organisms such as the stallion to enable the androgenizing effects of the male hormones. She provides an elaborate account that turns on the fact that the disproportionate interest in female sex hormones was due to the existence of a gynecological medical tradition (versus an andrological one) that dichotomized the process of knowledge production around these molecules. Her approach is important because it demonstrates that endocrine sex does not reflect a natural order of things but was, and indeed continues to be, produced by laboratory and clinical practices. Biologist and medical historian Anne Fausto-Sterling goes further in revealing the extent to which early endocrinologists operated with a heavily gendered understanding of sexual identity. She argues that "steroid hormones need not have been divided into sex and nonsex categories" (Fausto-Sterling 2000, 28). Doing so, she argues, has meant that "the signs of gender—from genitalia, to the anatomy of gonads and brains, then to our very body chemistry—[have been integrated] more thoroughly than ever into our bodies" (147). In this sense, Fausto-Sterling demonstrates that the chemical model of sex developed by endocrinology—and shaped by the gendered assumptions that orientated these early endocrinologists' work—actually drove the inscription of gender deeper and more pervasively into the body. The implication of this is twofold. First, it effectively sexes the *whole* body, including organs such as the brain, or behaviors that have come to be interpreted as indexes of sexual identity. Second, it obscures the far-reaching nonreproductive and nonsexual effects of steroid hormones by granting excessive attention to their sexual characteristics or by sexualizing their nonsex functions (Fausto-Sterling 2000).

In this chapter I explore a range of practices in which the gendered dimensions of hormones are foregrounded. My question concerns the homogeneous and ostensibly immutable representation of these complex—indeed, multiple—objects in Brazilian gynecological practices. As my attention turned toward more marginal hormonal practices, the possibilities afforded by hormones to challenge normative gender began to emerge. The unity of "multiple objects" follows from what Mol (2002) calls bracketing, namely the tendency to conceal the work of stabilization that goes into making objects appear as singularities—or natural kinds of a sort. Bracketing, or stating something *tout court*, obscures what Latour (1999, 190) calls the "blind spot in which society and matter exchange properties." The point here is simply to note that sex hormones only become part of discourse and agents in therapeutic relations when they are made to appear as discursive entities or laboratory materials (Oudshoorn 1994); that is, they need to be made knowable in particular ways in order to produce specific effects. What is remarkable is that laboratory life and medical practices bracket diversity, holding the different manifestations of sex hormones together as though they were all referring to one thing. In the end, this bracketed singularity is imagined as a piece of nature, as given. Yet, if we consider that work is required to signify bodily substances, physiological functions, and anatomical parts as indexes of fundamental sexual difference, and that this work is in turn concealed, then my aim here is to trace how hormones are called in to perform this task. In this process, my attention turns to what is going on at the margins and to how this may contribute to shaking the edifice of binary sex. I thus examine the extent to which the local idea of hormônio simply reinscribes sexual dimorphism, with estrogen emblematizing gendered activities and characteristics of femininity and testosterone signifying masculinity, and ask whether, in practice, hormônio exceeds such dichotomizations. I begin by exploring how hormonal practices that challenge normative sexual dimorphism and that can be considered forms of hormonal gender bending are presented or perceived in Bahia. Drawing on ethnographic and interview data with gynecologists, women, and *travestis* in Salvador, I propose that hormônio is understood as a kind of fluid or substance, not unlike blood. I build on the very specific material understandings of hormones to show how hormônio, like blood, is understood to have the capacity to accumulate in the body's cavities, producing growths or swellings. This opens the way for a discussion of hormônio as a gendered substance that, in its circulations, reveals an additional manner in which bodies are understood in Bahia to be plastic and malleable. I conclude by suggesting that local uses of pharmaceutical sex hormones and the diffusion, in Salvador, of medical ideas of hormonally produced gender cannot be reduced to a reinscription of sexual dualism. In this sense, prescribed and informal uses of these pharmacotherapies enact a troubling of both sex/gender and the distinction between them. Yet this occurs in a highly contested arena.

Circulating Sex Outside the Body

The question of how hormones are involved in the gendering of bodies dawned on me with particular force during the last month of an extended fieldwork period carried out in 2005 and 2006. I found myself dashing from one place to the next and traveling through radically different contexts with even greater intensity than previously. It is precisely this juxtaposition of contexts and the ensuing discussions that took place over the course of this particularly busy week that afforded the specific insights I hope to convey here. I had extended my stay in Salvador to attend the Brazilian Society for Gynecological Endocrinology Congress held in Salvador's luxurious Othon Palace hotel. In the run up to this event I was wrapping up other research avenues, and the evening before the congress began, I did the final part of an extensive life history with Manuela, a travesti, on her use of hormones.

Travestis adopt oral contraceptive pills, hormone replacement therapies, and hormonal contraceptive injections that they obtain in informal ways as part of their bodily transformation projects. Hormones designed for physiological females are used according to specific ideas about sexuality and embodiment and based on travesti hormone knowledge, which is detailed, exhaustive, and somewhat disregarding of adverse health effects. Homemade hormonotherapies of these kinds often double or triple the recommended dosages for physiological females, thus producing very blatant effects in their users. They are particularly appreciated for their effects in producing a feminine disposition and figure, in reducing bodily and facial hair, softening the voice, and changing the quality of the skin, and are said by travestis to quebrar o machão dentro da gente [break the macho inside us]. Travestis note their preference for injectable methods, referring to their milk color and quality, or evoking the nausea caused by the paste-like deposit that is said to accumulate in the stomach when hormones are ingested orally.

In the course of my interaction with ATRAS [behind], the tongue-in-cheek acronym chosen by the Travesti Association of Salvador, and given my interest in hormones, I was made aware of the political dimension of the struggle to obtain proper medical recognition and assistance. On one hand, the struggle involved securing access to basic health care; given the high levels of prejudice toward travestis (who are regularly assimilated to "prostitutes" and "marginals") and the disjunction between their physical appearance and the names on their identity documents, travestis often find themselves excluded from medical institutions. On the other hand, the struggle involved securing recognition of their specific medical needs and obtaining hormônio in the right dosage. Until recently there was no medical provision in the Brazilian public health sector for gender reassignment. Discussions were under way, and the official position seemed to be that should a medical protocol be established in Brazil, it should match existing protocols in North America and Europe, where hormone therapy for gender reassignment was dispensed only to individuals wishing to undergo genital surgery.[2] In 2009 the first outpatient service for travestis and transsexuals in Brazil was inaugurated in São Paulo (by the HIV/STD Reference Centre). Protocols in place include orientations and definitions of hormonal dosages for the development of so-called secondary sexual characteristics. According to the official press release made by the center six months after its inauguration, 45 percent of consultations were for hormonal therapies, 37 percent for sex-change surgery, and 14 percent for the removal of industrial silicone.[3] Manuela, an activist campaigning for travesti rights, explained to me in an interview[4]: "For us, hormônio is an inevitable evil. We have a feminine identity, we want to assume a feminine identity, but because of the prejudice in the medical perspective, hormonal therapies are only given to those who want to prepare themselves for surgery. We are here fighting for the right to be feminine, to have access to the necessary medical care to assume our identity, but without the obligation to undergo surgery, because we want to retain our penis."

This question came up many times in the weekly ATRAS meetings I attended. In one such meeting, the question of which medical specialist should be sought was raised. One person thought that a gynecologist would be most appropriate, given their knowledge of female hormones. She di-

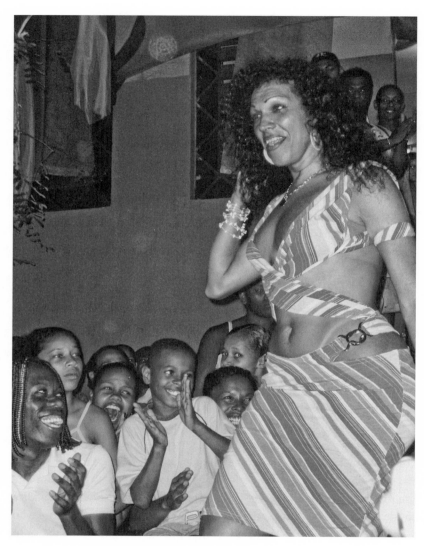

Figure 3.1 "Mrs." Paulo parading at ATRAS's (travesti association) sewing club's end-of-year fashion show with friends and family. Photograph by Emilia Sanabria.

rected the question to me but Natália, the chair, cut in, exclaiming, "Are you crazy?[5] What gynecologist? A gynecologist won't resolve anything! You don't have a uterus and ovaries, you have a prostate and testicles! What gynecologist is going to look after your prostate you crazy bitch?!"

This states the problem in its acute form, for in Salvador there is to this day no medical assistance for travestis, a fact that generates concerns about the informal uses travestis make of pharmaceutical hormones. For ATRAS this question has been singled out as one of political importance, a position that Manuela relayed to me in her commentary on her refusal to submit herself to the gender binary reproduced by biomedical practice, according to which individuals wishing to effect changes in their sexual identity must do so entirely, so to speak, or not at all. As a result, she explained, travestis make use of hormones in a completely improvised manner, raising substantial concerns regarding the long-term effects of this practice on their health.

My meeting with Manuela finished late that evening, and the next morning I walked into the first panel of the Gynecological Endocrinology Congress entitled: "The Use of Androgens in Gynecology," presided over by Elsimar Coutinho. This was a very official affair, including the Congress's opening address, drawing TV cameras and a large conference hall entirely packed. The panel members presented the different types of subdermal hormonal implants currently available, their composition and clinical use. In lauding these hormonotherapies and in speaking to an audience concerned primarily with the clinical aspects of treatment, the discussants moved seamlessly through biochemistry, gender politics, and risk management. The testosterone presentation given by Elsimar Coutinho was immediately followed by the screening of a documentary produced for Britain's Channel 4 and entitled: "Testosterone: Are you Man Enough?" This documentary explores the uses made of testosterone by both men and women, not only as a treatment for declining libido but also, increasingly, as a means of boosting assertiveness and self-confidence. A condensed version of the narration is reproduced here[6]:

> Narration: Imagine a drug that made you younger, richer, sexier, and all you had to do was rub it on. . . . It's the fastest growing smart drug, with sales topping $200 million. . . . The testosterone revolution is coming. Will you be able to resist? . . .
>
> Nick Neave: I think that testosterone is a hidden force that shapes our society, whether we like it or not. . . .

Dr. Tedde Rinker, Anti-ageing specialist: I call testosterone the yes hormone....

Jeff Lammert: It starts with a rush. It's like a rush of hotness throughout your body, not hot as in sweat, hot as it's coming from the core of your body. And it's a complete rush. The next day, I notice the change, there's a bit more spring in my stride. My mind was clearer ...

Narration: There are well-documented cases now of prostate cancer in younger people who've been taking high levels of testosterone, and there's also quite good evidence of increase in fat levels in the blood. We've certainly seen heart attacks and premature death.

Pierre Bouloux: More and more middle-aged men are gambling with their health to reclaim a bit of youth.

Narration: But menopausal men are just the tip of the iceberg. Europe's most radical hormone specialist is asking, why wait to get old? ... Herthoghe is 45. He's been self-medicating testosterone for 15 years ... Herthoghe believes the male hormone could even help cut the divorce rate. He claims to have rescued relationships with testosterone alone.

Dr. Thierry Herthoghe: I think that a lot of couples that want to divorce because of sex problems, or low love problems, are just hormone deficient persons ...

Narration: Testosterone isn't for men only. Its most dramatic effect is as an aphrodisiac for women....

Dr. Thierry Herthoghe: My wife takes testosterone, I have a sister who takes testosterone. Even my mother takes small doses of testosterone....

Narration: It's the most surprising aspect of the testosterone revolution. Women are taking it too, and seeing the world through men's eyes.

Grace Ross: The fact that I take testosterone helps me understand, I think, has given me more insight on how men think, and I can understand why they think about sex all the time....

Narration: Yes, testosterone makes you feel sexy, but it also makes you feel powerful.

Malcolm Whitehead, Gynecologist: I have patients who may have started testosterone because of poor sexual response, but they realize that the major benefit to them is the psychological boost they get in terms of being able to cope more effectively in a male dominated environment.

Claude Mahaux: I take testosterone when I have to act like a man. It's amazing to see how you can be like a man for a few hours, and to stay a real woman after.... The world is so demanding to us, you know, we have a life in our—with our family, we have a life with our husband, work, leisure, sex, it's so many different activities, and testosterone gives you maybe the power and energy to put your limits in all these little domains....

Narration: Until now, extra testosterone has been a luxury for the rich and powerful. Not anymore. US prescriptions for the drug are doubling each year, and like Viagra, a booming black market makes it readily available.... Once, natural selection put a cap on natural hormone levels, now we can cheat biology.

This was a very striking way to conclude a panel at a medical congress. During the question time that followed, Coutinho stood up, microphone in hand, and addressed the overflowing hall of gynecologists, medical students, and journalists, transforming what might have been a more scientifically informed discussion into a statement about "the patient's right to choose." Such a formulation clearly reveals the tension between what Mol (2008) has called the logic of choice and the logic of care in health. "'Woman,'" Coutinho solemnly announced, "can now be *dona* [mistress] of her own body and no longer needs to subject herself to the 'rules' established by society." Such a statement was meant as a pun, as in Portuguese the word for rule (*regra*) is the same as the word for menstrual period. He continued, asking us to imagine—in the subjunctive, throughout—that his good friend Marta Suplicy, the recently remarried mayor of São Paulo, had come to him and asked him for something that would give her a bit of *fogo* (fire)[7] for her honeymoon. Pausing, frowning, and cocking his head to the side, he asked his partly enchanted, partly skeptical audience:

What is one to do? Refuse it [testosterone] to her on the basis of a few potential and ill-explored risks? Tell her: "No Marta, stop being silly. What do you think a woman of your age is doing taking on the largest city in Latin America? Go back to your grandchildren and your knitting, and what's this business about honeymoons? You're too old for that nonsense." Is that what you would have me tell her? No my friends, I will not do that. But if you want to adopt that attitude, that's fine, but don't tell your patients that it can't be done, tell them *you* won't do it and send them to us here at CEPARH![8]

Taken together, these cases illustrate that while sex hormones seem to be reproducing sexual dimorphism, in the manner in which they are coded as female and male, when we turn specifically to an analysis of their uses, something else is revealed. Indeed, androgens (such as testosterone) may now be summoned with no apparent contradiction for patients or doctors in the making of new forms of femininity. With testosterone, women can be like men and yet remain women, we are told. They can become superwomen. Super-desiring and desirable. And perhaps, above all, super-productive. The cases above illustrate that inasmuch as hormones are produced as pharmaceutical drugs, the sexing of bodies is now at least partially exogenous to the body. The specific practices described here, although somewhat marginal still, are suggestive of the potential for gender bending that the circulation of hormones affords. Hormones—in their local and fluid manifestation as hormônio—have come to be understood as a kind of substance that circulates between bodies, producing gendering effects. While the transmutation of male substance into female bodies is medically and socially legitimated, the contrary is not true. This recontextualization of hormônio as a kind of substance has two sets of implications for what I have been referring to here as the plasticity of the body in Bahia. The first concerns the relative plasticity of sex/gender as the different aspects of what are commonly held to make up sex (e.g., specific genitalia or bodily characteristics) and gender (e.g., appearance, behavior) become dissociated from bodies and, in the form of pharmaceutical drugs, creams, gels, pills, injections, and so on, can now be absorbed from an exogenous source, conferring new identities. The second, which I attend to below, concerns the ideas my informants commonly hold about bodily fluids and substances and their transmutations. Hormônio, like blood, obeys a hydraulic logic in local understandings of the body. Interventions are seen to affect the quality or modify the flow of these fluids, demonstrating an understanding of the body as inherently malleable and actively partaking in its transformation.

The Fluid Properties of Hormônio

The meaning of the term hormônio, which I encountered daily during fieldwork in Salvador, is not fully captured by the English term hormone, although this was the term that I found myself using. As in English, hormônio commonly refers to the physiological hormones produced by the body, responsible for the menstrual cycle, *desejo* [sexual desire], *raiva* [rage], or *irritabilidade* [irritability]. While men and women have hormônio, it is mostly elaborated on in reference to "female hormones." Similarly, *hormônio* also refers to a class of drugs that include both *anticoncepcional* (the generic term for hormonal contraceptives) and *reposição* (literally, replacement), such as in the case of hormone replacement therapy (HRT). However, *hormônio* exceeds the standard meanings of the English term *hormone* because it occupies a semantic gap opened by humoral ideas about bodily capacities, which in Brazil are narrated as deriving from seventeenth-century versions of Hippocratic medicine that were brought to Brazil by European physicians. This humoral understanding of bodies is based on ideas about the flow and transmutability of substance and is one in which a body's plasticity and susceptibility to internal or extraneous transformations are assumed.

Women I interviewed across different social classes spoke as readily of taking hormônio as of taking the pill. For example, it was common for people to speak of taking "a" hormônio in reference to individual pills. When referring to hormonal levels (monitored as part of the widespread use of HRT) women would make comments such as *"minha taxa de hormônio 'ta otima"* (my hormone level is fine), or say: *"o medico falou que o meu hormônio caiu"* (the doctor said that my hormone [level] fell). Doctors and medical professionals engaged in gynecology and family planning, in discussions they have together, refer almost solely to the active principles and dosages, rather than to the myriad of brand names that exist for any given association of hormones.[9] When addressing patients, however, they often adopt the language they attribute to them and make statements along the lines of *"Você ta se dando bem com o hormônio?"* (Are you getting on OK with the hormone?) or *"Volte com seu preventivo e seus hormônios"* (Come back with your smear test and your hormones [levels]). On the other hand, pharmacists and pharmaceutical laboratory representatives speak generically of hormônio and introduced me to each other as doing research on hormônio. The common usage, in Bahia, of the singular form gives it a fluid, homogenous quality that is absent in the plural form. Further, the most commonly reported effects of hormônio are weight gain and swelling (*inchaço*), which reinforces the idea of hormônio as a very material substance that comes to saturate the body, filling its cavities. In this rendering, hormônio retains fluid-like properties rather than coming to be understood—as might be expected in such a medicalized context—as a class of entities with causal properties, as implied by the notion of chemical messengers. This question of terminology and semantic content emerged with particular clarity in the answers that the ill-designed question on hormones in my question guide received. I had included a targeted question on hormones that turned out somewhat to inhibit people's responses rather than stimulate the hormonal narrative I had imagined. The question was: "If you had to explain to someone how hormones work, what would you say?," and I would often add pointers to the effect of "based on your experience" or "how they are involved in the menstrual cycle." The question did not work at all in the way I had anticipated, and while my other questions seemed to fit, at least superficially, with local framings of the issues they broached, there was a clear ambiguity here that struck me as particularly revealing. Women often felt caught out by the question. On the other hand, I found that travestis answered much more comfortably, less concerned with being perceived as "ignorant." Within the divided social landscape of Salvador, the metaphors through which people understand and narrate their bodies' capacities and workings vary substantially. These social differences are (re)made through medical understanding and compliance to medical regimes. Middle-class patients tend to hold more closely to authoritative images and reveal a concern with accurate medical knowledge that is explained by the way in which *ignorancia* (ignorance) or *crendices* (beliefs)—as medical professionals refer to them—themselves become class attributes. Today, ignorance about medical regimes continues to index social marginality and poverty, and being *esclarecido* (knowledgeable) about the body is key to being recognized as a "modern," urban subject. Generally, the question, "How do hormones work?" was met with an answer about the clinical effects of pharmaceutical hormones, such as weight gain, headaches, or swelling. I would then push the question further, asking about the relation between these kinds of hormones and the hormones in the body, or about how hormones produced the effects that were so regularly attributed to them, but this would generally be met with silence. Part of the issue comes from the inclusion of the reference to experience in the question. This indicates that experience is understood to refer to clinical symptoms, to knowledge about the relation between the drug and the effects in the body. Experience does not capture the world of how people explain to themselves how hormones work. For example, Antonia, a nurse working in a plastic surgery clinic who has been using Depo-Provera as a treatment for endometriosis for over ten years, answered my question about hormonal action with reference to the effects Depo-Provera had on her body.

People generally say they are afraid of gaining weight and many people do put on weight when they take hormônio. But I didn't feel anything, no change whatsoever. On the contrary, my life changed for the better. There was no disadvantage in not menstruating. Except that it took me three years to get pregnant because of the hormônio. . . . I wouldn't know how to speak of the action, I can speak about advantages, but the action itself, you caught me out there! I'm not very curious with those things, I trusted my doctor because he is my uncle.

Rosedete is twenty-seven and was prescribed Implanon (a contraceptive hormonal implant produced by Organon) by her gynecologist, who did not, however, explain to her that this method is hormonal.

He only said it was this thing you put under the skin, barely bigger than a match. I didn't know anything [about it] but then I didn't really ask. I only discovered it was hormonal when I saw the effects. As the months went by I started to put on a lot of weight. Because if I stopped using Depo-Provera because of the weight gain, how is it that I would have put the implant in knowing it was hormônio? The doctor said I needed to "close my mouth" [fechar boca] because it is food, not hormônio, that causes weight gain. I know the weight gain is from the hormônio because I only started to gain weight when I started using hormônio. I don't understand how hormônio functions in my body, mais que age? Age! [but it sure does act!]

Tatiana, a journalist I interviewed, answered the question of how hormones work by talking about the pleasure and relief afforded by the flux of the menstrual blood. Moving seamlessly from this phenomenological account of menstrual bleeding to hormônio, she said: "I wanted to know more about that hormonal thing, so I put 'pineal' into Google. Apparently it's a portal of connections . . ." I pushed the hormonal question a little further and she answered: "I don't know anything about hormônio! I wouldn't even know where to start. . . . I don't even know what those bichinhos [little things/ animals] are called!" Similarly, Nanda, a communications consultant who had lived in the United States for several years, answered the question of how hormones work in the following way:

I see the function of hormônio in women, the oscillation of hormônio, as if it was the antithesis of the rational. Funny that way of seeing, isn't it? The hormonal person is completely surrendered, subject to the body, and does things that they don't want to rationally, loses control. Woman is a being completely full of hormônio, and has to deal with that. With menstruation, I feel renewed. I don't think it's dirty, but I have the sensation of cleansing, evacuation, that it comes out because it has to come out. Why would you have all that accumulated up there? But I'm talking like a lay person now.

The immediacy of the association in these statements between hormones and the relief afforded by menstrual bleeding is striking and came up with great regularity in the course of fieldwork. As my attention grew away from menstruation and came to concern how people make sense locally of the notion of hormônio, I initially failed to recognize the significance of my informants' talk about blood in response to my questions about hormones.

Hormônio, Blood, and Substance

In Bahia, then, hormônio is understood as a kind of substance, not unlike blood itself in certain respects. Hormônio and blood are alike principally because both of these materials are understood to have the capacity of accumulating in the body, lodging themselves within the body's cavities and producing discomfort, swelling, or growths. These understandings were revealed to me through ethnographic work I had the opportunity of carrying out in Salvador's blood donation center, Hemoba. I made contact with the blood donation staff after several interviewees made explicit connections between menstruation, blood donation, and bloodletting, evoking the physical alleviation procured by the act of giving blood (for further details see Sanabria 2009). Patients at the blood donation center at times adopted blood donation as a means of dispelling the discomfort caused by what they referred to as *sangue grosso* ["thick" blood]. Thick blood is understood to cause itching of the skin, dizziness, and a sense of discomfort or pins and needles. Women are seen not to need to donate blood as much as men, who, in the absence of menstruation, are more prone to thick blood and require a means to expunge the ensuing excess. While thick blood tends to result from an accumulation of blood or the consumption of "strong" foods (such as Bahian foods, which are rich in palm oil), the use of hormones is also evoked by blood donation patients as leading to blood disturbances.

Bahian notions of *sangue* (blood) are central to understandings of how bodies are internally constituted and influenced by exogenous sources of different kinds. In many of my informants' perspectives, sangue does not obey the same rules as the capillary blood described by Western anatomy. The state and the quality of sangue are in constant transformation, affected by the types of foods eaten as well as by the climate, strong emotions, physical activity, or practices of purification or purging. These factors can render sangue *grosso* (thick) or *fino* (thin). While sangue grosso tends to stagnate in the body, obstructing the circulation of energy, sangue fino does not sustain the organism enough and leaves a person without *animo* (energy/vitality). Sangue is thus a trope through which people convey ideas of lassitude, bodily capacities, well-being, or emotion. This humoral understanding of bodies is based on ideas about the flow and transmutability of substance, and is one in which a body's plasticity and susceptibility to internal or extraneous transformations are assumed. Exogenous influences, such as climatic forces or the intentions and feelings of others, such as *mal olhar* (evil eye) and *olho grosso* (jealousy), may affect sangue, causing physical disturbances in the person upon whom they fall. In Afro-Brazilian traditions, *axé*, the life force, circulates through sangue (blood). Axé can be absorbed, wasted, or accumulated, and all personal accomplishments are dependent on the proper management of axé. Generally speaking, in Bahia—that is, beyond strictly Afro-Brazilian religious contexts—blood is closely associated with strength. Sangue must circulate in a state of balance to confer strength. Its excessive accumulation or an unbalance of sangue is debilitating and considered pathological. These older, humoral conceptions are transformed and reinforced through contemporary biomedical discourses around the management of blood, such as those pertaining to diabetes, hypertension, cardiovascular disease, or menstrual suppression.

The main manner in which hormônio is understood to act on blood is through its effects on the flow of menstrual blood. This in turn indicates that arterial and menstrual blood flows are intrinsically connected rather than radically dissociated, as is often the case according to the ethnographic literature on menstruation and menstrual taboos (e.g., Buckley and Gottlieb 1988). In Bahia—where, as we have seen, many women have at one time or another experimented with hormones to suppress menstrual bleeding—the question of what happens to menstrual blood when it is not evacuated is subject to diverse interpretations. Marilene is a nursing auxiliary who works at the Hemoba and is herself a regular blood donor. One afternoon I sat talking with her at a table in the snack bar adjacent to the donation room, where I would collect patients' testimonies after they had donated blood. Explaining my research to her, I relayed that many of the women interviewed as part of my research on menstruation said they enjoyed the freedom of not menstruating procured by the use of certain hormonal regimes but express concerns about the blood accumulating. "I agree, you know. That blood has to be expulsed. I see a necessity for that. I know a person who put on a lot of weight, whose abdomen was distorted because of this [menstrual suppression]. And really, in her case, it's visible, she uses that injection [Depo-Provera] to stop menstruating. I hate menstruating but I don't do that. If I had a problem, a uterine fibroma or that kind of thing, I would remove my uterus [have a hysterectomy]. But to arrest all that blood there [in the uterus], never."

On this occasion, a patient came out of the donation room and, hearing our conversation, joined in: "I take Depo-Provera injections because I hate menstruating.... The injection is good. Many women still have a taboo with the injection.... Many people don't like Depo-Provera but they don't know what they are missing. I used Microvlar, but it made me nauseous, to take pills every day. Depo-Provera was my salvation. When I stop taking it, I will *estrangular* [literally, "strangle," a popular term for tubal ligation]."

Drawing on the trope of "usefulness" made popular by Coutinho's book *Menstruation: Useless Bleeding*, Joseneide then added—half seriously, half in jest—that the advantage of giving blood was that "at least when you donate blood, this blood [unlike menstrual blood] is useful to someone and not just wasted!" I was struck by Joseneide's ingenious approach to menstrual suppression. She then explained to us that she had been diagnosed with a uterine fibroid, which she says the scan revealed to be as large as her fist. As a long-term Depo-Provera user, she understands the fibroid to be the result of hormônio accumulating in her uterus, forming the growth. Although in Brazil most doctors opt for a surgical treatment of fibroids (and in many cases hysterectomy), the last doctor she saw prescribed a hormonal treatment to reduce the size of the uterine growth. Joseneide is wholly unconvinced by this approach, given that she understands hormônio accumulation to have produced the growth in the first place. She is actively seeking a hysterectomy and jokes that for women who already have children, the uterus is *descartável* (disposable), a phrase one commonly hears in Bahia. Given that I have been asked to wear a lab coat by the blood donation staff, Joseneide asks me whether I can find her a doctor who will recommend a hysterectomy, as the doctor in her local health post has refused her request. In her narrative, contraception (as in "strangulating," or surgical sterilization), prophylactic hysterectomy, and the iatrogenic origin of her fibroid blend seamlessly, suggesting that the popularity of surgical procedures in Bahia may in part have their origin in local conceptualizations of humoral accumulation: "Do you know if instead of 'strangulating,' there is a doctor who could just take my uterus out and be done with it? Because I always say: 'the uterus only serves for three things: menstruating, having children and getting disease.' My mother had a hidden fibroid, you know. It seems that after you menstruate [menopause], when it stops, then the hormônio accumulates. I think when you strangle [sterilize], then menstruation accumulates — I don't really know why — and then it [the uterus] augments. Hormônio gives fibroids, right? So why not just remove the uterus straightaway?"

This case reveals the close association of ideas of swelling and pathological accumulation (in the form of the uterine fibroid) associated with the retention of both blood and hormônio. This blood donation patient resolved the problem of menstrual suppression in an extraordinary way, dispelling both the inconveniences of menstrual bleeding and its swelling effects by turning to a further medical intervention: blood donation. However, this action — and the accompanying notion of giving the otherwise useless menstrual blood a positive and altruistic function — has not resolved the problem of hormônio accumulation, to which she attributes the appearance of her fibroid. In taking up this strategy she effectively separated hormônio from blood and reproduced the problem in a different form. These brief ethnographic examples drawn from work with blood donors reveal that hormônio is often conceptualized in humoral terms in Bahia. Like blood, it is subject to pathological accumulation, and interventions (often surgical in nature) are required to redress an unbalance in this "humor." What is striking about these examples is that they reveal that the body is understood as a kind of recipient-like enclosure or container that can be filled and purged. These actions in turn have implications for the ontological status of bodies. They show that bodies are not experienced as entirely fixed and immutable. While the tangible materiality of biological inscriptions is widely recognized, this is not to be taken as permanent or finished.[10] Rather, bodies are open to modification and perpetually in becoming. As we have seen here, actions on the status and quality of blood, or on the flow of hormônio, may radically transform bodies. In this sense they reveal a further facet of what I am underscoring here as the plasticity and malleability of the body in Bahia.

The anthropological literature on substance is vast and has a complex historiography (Carsten 2011) that I will not rehearse here. For the present purposes, I would simply like to draw attention to the way in which, in a range of contexts, transmutations in bodily substances such as blood, semen, milk, or menstrual blood are understood to produce differences in the sexual capacities or attributes of persons. The analogies or asymmetric evaluations made between different bodily substances are at the basis of many gender systems (see Gregor and Tuzin 2001; Héritier 1996; Mosko 1985; and Strathern 1988). These understandings flow from a widespread understanding that, while being associated with one or the other gender, substances are transformable and transmutable between bodies. For example, among the Samo of Burkina Faso, as described by Héritier, semen is understood to turn into blood in a woman's body (blood that she loses during menstruation). Godelier (1996) accounts for what he sees as the ideological domination of Baruya women in New Guinea by reference to the way bodily substances are conceived. He shows that for the Baruya, breastmilk is in fact understood to be semen. Strathern (1988, 1991, 1992b) outlines this asymmetry rather differently. Characteristically, she shows that the substances in and of themselves cannot, as Godelier's analysis suggests, be thought of as attributing sexual identity. Rather, they mediate particular relations that are themselves gendered.[11] As she argues, the power of these substances lies precisely in the fact that they are transferable between persons. Strathern (1988) powerfully reveals how, in Melanesia, gender is not an attribute of a body but rather of relations that involve the detachment, elicitation, or exchange of substances. Carsten (2011) shows how the term *substance* has been used to do quite different things in anthropological theorizations of kinship and the body. She points first to the multiple meanings this notion has within the English language: as essence; separate distinct thing; that which underlies phenomena; or corporeal matter. This polysemy in part explains how the term *substance* was effectively taken up to signify divergent meanings. Within analyses of Western conceptions of kinship—such as in the work of Schneider (1980)—substance (and blood, in particular) came to stand for that which is unalterable and indissoluble. On the other hand, Carsten shows the term was adopted in Indian and Melanesian ethnography to speak of the mutability and fluidity underpinning notions of the person.

So how is the term *substance* useful to explain Bahian understandings of hormônio? In drawing attention to the fluid properties of both hormônio and blood, my intention is first and foremost to attend to the ethnographic questions that ideas about blood and hormônio raise. These reveal an idea of bodies as relatively undifferentiated enclosures, which can be filled or purged of their excesses. Such interventions in turn have effects on the onto-logical status of bodies, both transforming what, in other contexts, is seen as immutable biology, and thereby disturbing "the" body as a sign of such facts of nature. Blood, like hormônio, is to some extent foundational to a person's identity in a manner that is cognate with biological understand-ings. However, these are not understood to confer identities that are fixed or immutable, as the many examples given above demonstrate. In the final section, I trace the implications this has for the question of sexual dimor-phism with which I opened.

One-Sex Thinking in the Two-Sex World

Perhaps the most telling lay interpretation of hormones came from tra-vesti exegeses, expounded of the course of the weekly ATRAS meetings I attended. On one occasion, the chair had introduced me as an anthropolo-gist working on hormônio. She asked the participants whether they would be willing to talk about their experiences with hormônio, and to detail both the use they had made of different drugs and the positive or adverse effects these had produced. Commentary flowed freely, and many travestis spoke of their experience with these drugs in terms of being *cheia* (full, in the femi-nine) of hormônio. This is illustrated most clearly by the striking image of hormônio oozing at the place where it is injected. Several travestis noted that, at the time when they had most injected contraceptives, their bodies were so full of hormônio that it would drip from the place of the injection, like a fluid that has reached the watermark. This explicit statement about the substance-like nature of hormônio both informs and is informed by other statements about hormônio, such as an example given by Kulick (1998, 66), which points to the transmutability of hormônio-as-substance in travesti exegesis: "travestis also believe that it is unwise for them to ejaculate while they are taking hormones, because they think that hormones are expelled from the body in that way. Each ejaculation, therefore, means progressively smaller breasts."

During one particularly memorable weekly meeting of the travesti asso-ciation, a lively debate arose regarding the use of different brands to grow breasts. Breasts are often born out of repeated hormonal injections, and tra-vestis commonly speak of using hormônio to *tomei hormônio para fazer nascer meu peito* [give birth to breasts]. Hormones are used before the "pumping" of liquid industrial silicone because they are said to mold and shape the body from the inside, giving rise to a form that can later be filled with liquid industrial silicone.[12] Latent within this debate about which hormones best produced breasts were tensions surrounding issues of identity politics of which I was not yet fully aware. One member of the group, Marlene, stated that, "My chest is [é] Depo-Provera," a comment that echoes the statement that someone's breasts "are" silicone (e.g., *seu peito é silicone*). This rendition reinforces the idea of hormones as a kind of material that is understood quite literally to fill the body. The tension rose when Marlene continued, specifying that when she injected herself regularly with Depo-Provera, her body had been so imbued with hormônio that her breasts had oozed with milk. Drawing out her pointy breast from under her shirt in a dramatic and defiant gesture and holding it in one hand she exclaimed: "I was so full of hormônio that my breasts *pingava leite* [dripped with milk]." At this point one of the other group participants cut in and exclaimed: "That wasn't milk, you crazy bitch, that was sperm!"

Marlene, with whom I subsequently carried out an interview, later gave me the context within which to understand this exchange afresh. She explained to me that, unlike the others, she was transsexual and not a travesti, a fact that earned her the stigmatization that had been obvious at the meeting, but the cause of which had been unclear for me. Unlike the travestis, whom she described as whorish and outrageous, she dressed in smart, office-like clothing. Her challenger was a stout, scathing, and highly sexual character who worked and lived "in the street" and for whom Marlene's effeminate manner lacked the edge her challenger unambiguously brought to the meetings. This challenge to Marlene's proud assertion of (full) femininity—breasts dripping with milk—through the reassertion of her concomitant masculinity, emblematized by sperm, illustrates the way in which hormônio is adopted to speak of bodily capacities to transmute fluids. The religious tenor of the story itself, in evoking an exuding miracle (such as the miraculous lactation of icons of the Virgin), common in Latin American Catholicism, reveals something of the potency of religious imagery in the definition of gendered norms. In alluding to the image of the nursing Virgin, Marlene is claiming for her own a specific representation of the feminine that is at odds with the highly sexualized representation to which other ATRAS meeting participants aspire.

Konrad's (1998) analysis of substance in Melanesian ethnography and among British ova donors provides suggestive material for comparison. She uses Melanesian ethnography to create a perspective from which to explore both contemporary and Renaissance notions of gender, sex, and body. Throughout the article she negotiates this set of contrasts to arrive at the conclusion that versions of the ideas of partibility and corporeal permeability are "in some sense indigenous to the Western canon of the human reproductive body" (659). The comparability of pre-Enlightenment ideas concerning bodily substances as residues of the differential heat in male and female bodies and Melanesian data on the transmutability of substances are convincingly demonstrated. However, the ethnography she presents from British ova donors seems to stretch her analysis a little thin at times. Konrad invites us to think about how activities of rechanneling substance have wider implications for the question of gender as it relates to the production of sociality. The paper is concerned with explaining how British ova donors perceive the process of superovulation.[13] Extracting ova requires both the interruption of menstruation and the absorption of synthetic hormones. The process of taking hormones to stimulate ovulation is understood by the ova donors Konrad interviewed as simply replacing, pharmaceutically, what is lacking. She speaks of this as inducing a supersized femininity in the women by "adding more femaleness" (659). This "adding more" of one gender is made possible through the circulation of sex(ed) hormones, as we have seen in the proposal to use testosterone in hormonal regimes designed for physiological females or in the unofficial use travestis make of what they refer to as hormônio feminino (female hormones, or hormones traditionally prescribed to women). Returning to the comparison between Melanesia and Euro-America that Konrad sets out, however, one might ask whether the exteriorized ova of her analysis can in fact serve the purpose of illuminating the one with the other. How readily do they travel between the two contexts she sets out? Konrad is at times forced to make connections — such as between the donated ova and the arrested blood flow — that her informants themselves do not make. The Bahian material I present here can in a way mediate the analytic leap Konrad makes by supporting her proposition that the manner in which people engage with reproductive interventions and pharmacotechnologies can be seen as "local version[s] of concocting gender" (650). Departing from Konrad's paper, I have asked about the kinds of gender identities that are caught, so to speak, between the sexual binaries still dominant in biomedical practice and the possibilities that, in Salvador, are being explored by the rechanneling of "sexual substances." The flexibilization of genders, operated through redirected flows of hormônio that I have evoked here, seems geared toward the stabilizing of the body in particular socially desirable states: emotionally stable (versus unstable and hysterical), desiring, and competitive. But as we have seen already, practices that stabilize bodies inherently assume its malleability, as the intervention is geared toward bodily fixity or integrity, but this state is achieved only through intervention.

Konrad's British case stands in contrast to the Bahian one developed here in various ways, but the notion of substance made exogenous and circulating is operative in both and, as Konrad has shown can be fruitfully put to work against classical anthropological analyses of the transmutability of bodily substances. Her approach is useful in that it points to the way reproductive biotechnologies (be they those of assisted reproduction or the hormonal practices I describe here) produce a disjunction between (sexed) substance and sexed body. This notion of a rechanneling of sexual substances is further illustrated by an ethnographic instance that reveals a highly idiosyncratic Judeo-Christian origin to the idea of substance transmutation. Speaking of the importance of estrogen in clinical practice, one prominent female gynecologist addressed the aforementioned Gynecological Endocrinology Congress in the following manner:

> Estradiol is the feminine soul, it is estradiol that gives us the capacity to attract males. It is a fundamental hormônio. And I will add that testosterone without estradiol is nothing! Just as Eve came out of Adam's rib, estradiol is synthesized out of testosterone. It is a hormônio that no one notices, because it is so physiological. We women have had our era of reclusion, we were the property of the husband, then we had to be *macho* [male]. Now we can be more competitive, mothers, professionals, *and* feminine. Women today want an improvement in sexuality, and self-confidence. . . . So E2 brings back the position that women want, it is a very old hormone but it is very modern. It combines femininity and activity. (Dra Conzuelo)

Aside from revealing the powerful implications this has for understanding the hierarchical valuation of different hormones and the genders they effect, this statement reveals that—for this influential doctor, at least—we are well within the confines of what historian Thomas Laqueur calls the "one-sex" world. In his history of the making of sex, Laqueur (1990) showed that before the Enlightenment, discussions about the bodily basis of gender were "understood analogically" and based in metaphysics rather than empirical verification. He qualifies this period as one in which a "one-sex" model prevailed. In this model, two gendered bodies were derived from one single, paradigmatic, nonsexed body. Until this point, bodily facts did not, he argues, lend themselves to the same kind of ideological investment as they did with the advent of the new empirically based anatomy. It is in this latter context that the markedly different two-sex world emerged. Laqueur's model has been the subject of a great deal of valuable criticism (on the specificities of the transition from a one-sex to a two-sex model or on the existence of one-sex thinking in the two-sex world and vice versa), but for the purpose of this discussion I propose to hold on to the distinction he proposes, as a heuristic. Importantly, Laqueur demonstrates that the categories of "male" and "female" were more permeable and open to change through the intracorporeal channeling of sexual substances. Whether the female or the male be understood as the paradigm or the instance in this one-sex model, the point remains that difference, before the Enlightenment, was not "grounded in radically different sexual bodies" (Laqueur 2003, 305). The model Laqueur proposes is therefore useful, precisely because it provides a frame that reveals more clearly the phenomena that do not neatly fit into it. Hormônio, in the context I researched, clearly troubles the contemporary version of the two-sex model. This raises an issue that reaches beyond that of sexual dimorphism, concerning bodies, their capacities, and the biological ascription of limits to these capacities. What is interesting in Laqueur's model is that it sets out two extremes, and from the perspective of either of these, specific problems arise. In the one-sex model, the sharpness of observed sexual difference must be accounted for, and gave medieval writers — it seems — a great deal of worry (see Bynum 1991). On the other hand, from the perspective of the two-sex model that now occupies biomedical theories, the lability of sex and the shades of sexual difference arise as explanatory problems. In the context at hand, where the relationship between genitally determined sex and gendered possibilities is constantly being reworked, this is particularly blatant.

Reassembling Sex

"How do tacit normative criteria form the matter of bodies?" This is a question that philosopher Judith Butler (1993, 54) poses in Bodies That Matter. Butler's emphasis on the performative aspects of gender in Gender Trouble (1988) was critiqued for its disavowal of the constraints imposed by "sex." Bodies That Matter (1993) specifically attends to the ways in which norms material-

ize the body. In that historical analysis of the philosophy of matter, Butler shows that materiality is itself sexed. She describes "sex" as a *process* of materialization: "As a sedimented effect of a reiterative or ritual practice, sex acquires its naturalized effect, and, yet, it is also by virtue of this reiteration that gaps and fissures are opened up as the constitutive instabilities in such constructions, as that which escapes or exceeds the norm. . . . This instability is . . . the power that undoes the very effects by which 'sex' is stabilized" (10).

This chapter offers an ethnographic exploration into how sex hormones are implicated in specific "matterings" of bodies. Although hormones widely continue to be sexed in both scientific and popular imaginaries within a binary model of sex, the ethnographic materials presented here imply ways in which the reiteration of "sex" through hormonal practices is subject to the kinds of instabilities and excesses to which Butler calls attention.

Experiments with sex(ed) hormones produce identities that are difficult to account for in terms of sexual binaries, as the fascinating history of the sexing of steroid hormones and the ethnographic examples given here attest to. What is remarkable is the resilience of the binary system within which sex nevertheless continues to be understood. Consider the politics of naming among travestis, or the linguistic difficulties in describing the gender of a testosterone-boosted woman. In the hormonal practices mapped here, what is often evoked is the notion of adding—attaining a "feminine disposition" while retaining a penis, being "like a man" but staying a "real woman"—in the examples explored here. These facts point to what Fausto-Sterling has described as a sexing of the whole body through the chemical redefinition of sex. In a sense this can be seen to flow from the intricate connections that are drawn, both in scientific and in popular discourses, between anatomical structures, the "sex" that flows through the body's chemistry, and so-called secondary sexual characteristics or (sexed) behaviors. It is in this sense that I propose that prescribed and informal uses made of these pharmacotherapies enact a troubling both of sex/gender and of the distinction between them. As I have argued, the continuity between genital sex and the circulation of gender does not depend on the ineluctability of the facts of nature. Given the many biological and social elements that are required to make sex (and not just gender), efforts need to be constantly deployed to reassemble these with the consistency that makes us blind to the manufactured aspect of sex.

CHAPTER 4

HORMONAL BIOPOLITICS

FROM POPULATION CONTROL TO SELF-CONTROL

Biomedicine in Brazil is marked by unregulated overmedication and a predilection for surgical procedures, on the one hand, and by the absence of many basic services on the other. Access to medical services in this highly differentiated landscape of health provision thereby comes to be a key indicator of social differences. Public services are often overcrowded spaces where *atendimento* ("attention," wherein notions of care and cordiality mingle) is often described as harsh or rushed. Many doctors, who are faced with enormous queues each day, do not even look up from the forms in front of them at the patients. Here the language of patient rights may be inverted as patients are enjoined to fulfill their obligations as citizens by complying with biomedical regimes. A national policy for humanizing medical attention was launched in the mid-2000s. This sought to tackle physical and symbolic ill treatment and thus address the tension between the SUS's (public health) values of universality and the deeply hierarchical nature of Brazilian society. While the tangible effects of this policy are yet to be demonstrated, the term *humanização* has become a veritable buzzword, covering a heterogeneous set of concerns. Humanization is founded on the recognition of the patient's integrity and aims to equalize the structural inequalities of Brazilian society that are so starkly represented in access to health. The policy recognizes the social, cultural, and racial plurality of Brazilian society and identifies the problems of communication and information as central to the amelioration of health care. In late 2009 I carried out research on the polysemous meanings *humanização* carries in public health institutions. In the large health post on Avenida Carlos Gomes, which caters principally to a lower-middle-class population, a project on public perceptions of the impact of "humanizing" atendimento had been initiated by a social worker. Handwritten notes, many reading as grievance notes regarding the absence of drugs in the post's pharmacy or the difficulty in obtaining an appointment with a specialist, had been collected in a folder, which lay somewhat forlorn at the bottom of a metal drawer. One such note read as follows: "The receptionists are very rude. They act like we are asking for favors. It is nothing less than their obligation to attend to us. If they do not wish to do so, they should direct us to someone who will. Measures should be taken to humanize atendimento."

Private health insurance opens the doors to a very different set of medical institutions, which often place a premium on cordiality and the personalization of atendimento. Salvador boasts a series of prestigious glass-and-marble medical complexes, imaging and diagnostic laboratories, and renowned *consultórios* (private health practices). Accompanying doctors, who often work in both sectors, for example, attending in SUS *ambulatórios* in the morning and in their private consultórios in the afternoon, give a stark sense of the degree to which the services and treatment—as well as the spaces themselves—are highly differentiated. It makes clear the differences in the way hormonal contraceptives are administered to women of different backgrounds, highlighting the different goals underscoring both the choice of methods and the manner in which problems with specific methods are dealt with. Whereas in the SUS patients are treated in a highly standardized fashion, in these private institutions efforts are made to differentiate and personalize medical attention. Health care systems can be said to reflect larger social inequalities. Those reflected in Brazilian health services are particularly stark, however, encompassing extremes of both lavishness and want that are seldom observed together.

This chapter examines the highly differentiated ways in which public and private patients are treated in reproductive health services in Salvador. It traces practices of family planning and hormonal contraception prescription through a range of interconnected clinical contexts—including gynecological consultations, vasectomy clearance interviews, or postnatal care, where family planning is heavily emphasized—and institutional settings through which population data are administered. These structural differentiations can be traced all the way down to differences in the way sex hormones are differently packaged to distinct segments of the population. Sex hormones are widely adopted as strategies of intervention upon the population, in the context of national family planning policies, but they are also taken up to discipline subjectivities and enhance the self. Drawing on ethnographic descriptions of the processes of triage and negotiations of access to highly differentiated standards of care and atendimento, I initiate a broader discussion on health inequalities in Brazil through a critical discussion of the recent literature on biopolitics. I explore the implications that modes of differentiation in biomedical services have for the constitution of a public sphere in Brazil by tracing the range of publics that make up the Brazilian "collective." This reveals the way practices such as those at work in reproductive health create and reproduce what I call, following Brazilian anthropologist Roberto DaMatta, *sub-* and *super-*citizens.

Much of the literature on biopolitics recognizes the decline of disciplinary biopolitics and emphasizes a different kind of governance or management of the self. Somatic individuality, it is suggested, is increasingly important in the neoliberal political landscape (see, in particular, Rose 2007). However, the class dynamics underlying the social uses of medicine in Brazil differ from those in Britain or the United States, from where many of these analyses seem to be developed. Either these have a more equitable health care system or their clinical practices are more tightly regulated than they are in Brazil. As we have seen in previous chapters, remaking the body is considered *muito chique* (very chic) and key to renegotiating social hierarchies. Biomedicine is thus embroiled in aspirational class processes, where access to medical care of the kind associated with private medicine, to surgeries, and to imported pharmaceuticals is a means of literally embodying a form of class ascension. *Cuidar-se* (self-care) is not necessarily (just) about the self. It is also about making social relations through work on the body. Self-management—or, in the local idiom, cuidar-se—is thus frequently about taking care of relationships in ways that do not fit notions of neoliberal "self-governance" or "somatic individuality" (Edmonds and Sanabria 2014).

Differentiated Pharmaceutical Citizenships

Anthropological work on pharmaceuticals has shown that access to drugs (re)produces social differences. This is particularly true in the case of hormonal treatments and contraceptive methods, where a vast array of different brand names and modes of administration are available. Oudshoorn (1996) has argued that new technologies of hormonal administration differentiate between types of users who are deemed worthy of making individual choices and those whose fertility needs to be strictly controlled. Work shows how, historically, this shift responded to concerns with overpopulation in the Global South. In this chapter I show how these differences in how hormones are administered no longer map neatly onto North/South distinctions. These differentiations also operate *within* the national contexts, such as in Brazil, where both types of configured users are found.

In Brazil, as we have seen, hormonal contraceptives are administered in a variety of ways: both orally and nonorally. The modifications in dosages and forms of administration of sex hormones affect how these substances act in the body, that is, their bioavailability. My aim is to give an account of the way in which this class of pharmaceuticals is made available to women in the public and private health sectors according to quite distinct rationales. Second-generation oral contraceptives are widely distributed through the public health service and readily available in pharmacies for as little as R$5 per pack.[1] The more expensive third- and fourth-generation contraceptive pills are marketed through private practices in ways that reinforce the personalization of these hormonal treatments to women's "profile," age, and lifestyle and which tend to emphasize the drugs' effects in terms of well-being, weight loss, or aesthetics. Nonoral methods are widespread in Brazil and enjoy considerable media attention. These include trimonthly hormonal injections (such as Depo-Provera and its Brazilian "copy" Contracep), the hormone-releasing intrauterine system (Mirena[2]), and subdermal hormonal implants. Most of these methods intervene with regular menstruation, and with some methods menstruation ceases completely. As with oral methods, these vary widely in price, thus producing a range of configured users.[3] My interest here lies precisely at this intersection between the political and the pharmacological.

Two parallel forms of citizenship are revealed through an analysis of the kind of health care available in Brazil. In the context of reproductive health, the first — available to the privileged who can afford private health — is founded on notions of personal autonomy, individual choice, and self-enhancement, whereas the second frames reproductive decisions in terms of the individual's moral responsibility to the wider collectivity. Here, the regulation of bodies is closely assimilated to the regulation of the body of the nation. Patients are enjoined to fulfill their obligations as citizens. Ecks

(2005, 241) proposed the term *pharmaceutical citizenship* to consider how legal citizenship determines access to pharmaceuticals, on the one hand, and the implications of taking pharmaceuticals for a person's status as a citizen, on the other. For the urban poor, entering into medical regimes is a means of attaining a socially recognized status as a person, what Biehl (2004) refers to as "citizenship through patienthood." Being triaged, that is, is a means of demarginalization for it serves as an opportunity to be recognized and attended to by the state. As Tone (2001) and Murphy (2012, 16) have shown, the global project of family planning is a Cold War one: "With the pill given away as a form of foreign aid, the term nuclear family took a militarized turn."

Throughout the 1960s, and under the military dictatorship of Vargas, the Brazilian state adopted an explicitly pronatalist stance, a posture that evolved in the 1970s into what Bozon (2005, 362) refers to as a "socially selective Malthusianism" position targeting low-income women. Despite the fact that the Brazilian state never adopted a coherent set of policy instruments in favor of family planning, fertility rates plummeted between the mid-1960s and mid-1990s, from 5.7 children per woman to 2.3 for the country as a whole and 7.2 to 2.9 for the northeast. Bozon argues that this was an indirect effect of the medicalization of Brazilian society undertaken during the Vargas dictatorship, as well as of the rapid urbanization of the population and changing familial organization.[4] Similarly, Corrêa (2001, 56) showed that the medicalization of reproduction in Brazil was led by private-sector initiatives and international aid organizations, at times contrary to the official state position. Mapping the history of the pill's uptake in Brazil is difficult because it was not introduced as part of a planned public policy (Bozon 2005; Loyola 2010; Pedro 2003). The absence of a national family planning strategy created a void that was filled by the market that produced a contraceptive praxis characterized by drugstore-promoted self-medication. Enovid, the first pill to be introduced in Brazil, was promoted by salespersons in private gynecological practices and was available in pharmacies, although its cost was prohibitive for most (Pedro 2003). The pill was unevenly diffused among low-income women by the interventions of international nongovernmental organizations. This introduction of the pill via the market, rather than via the health system, gave rise to high rates of "ever use" and discontinuation, or what medical professionals refer to as "misuse" or "noncompliance." This can be explained by the fact that hormones circulate largely outside medical control and continue to be readily available over the counter, even without a prescription. In her oral history of the pill in Brazil, Pedro (2003) found that women recollected experiencing many discomforts with the pill, a fact that is mirrored in the media coverage that emphasized from the outset the risks and side effects of the initially highly dosed pills.

Nonoral hormonal methods, such as contraceptive injections, hormonal implants, or intrauterine hormonal devices like Mirena, are pitched by health care providers as efficient and reversible alternatives to sterilization, the rates of which remain uncharacteristically high in Brazil. This is reflected in the data on shifting patterns of contraceptive use in Brazil. According to a nationwide survey carried out in the mid-1990s, around 40 percent of women "aged 15–49 currently in a relationship" had undergone surgical sterilization (BEMFAM et al. 1996). In this study, hormonal injections accounted for only 0.8 percent of contraceptive methods used. A more recent survey (analyzed by Perpétuo and Wong 2009) estimated that the overall rate of female sterilization had gone down to around 25 percent, although significant disparities emerge when analyzing these figures according to level of education or economic class.[5] The study also reveals that 18.9 percent of women had at one time used hormonal contraceptive injections such as Depo-Provera, pointing to a relationship I wish to highlight here between declining rates of sterilization and rising rates of what are known in the international reproductive health community as "long-acting reversible contraceptive" methods (or LARCs). According to the most recent data, only 3.5 percent of women declare they are currently using the contraceptive injection. However, Perpétuo and Wong (2009, 100) conclude that: "Amongst women without education, injectable contraceptives were the second choice, closely behind female sterilization" (my translation). This can be explained by Depo-Provera being a cheap yet highly efficient, provider-administered method, a fact that is seen to overcome patient misuse associated with the use of the pill and guaranteeing contraceptive efficacy at a low cost. It tends to be widely administered to low-income women, without a discussion of health risks (particularly regarding bone mineral density), a fact that has raised concerns.[6]

In 1997, Pharmacia-Upjohn, which distributed Depo-Provera in Brazil, received $1 million from USAID to cut the price of Depo-Provera by 50 percent, thereby making it accessible to "lower-income consumers" while expanding "the potential market for the product," according to a UN report (UNFPA 1999, 28). Fort (2001, 22) reveals that Pharmacia-Upjohn was advised by the social marketing specialist Futures Group International to change their marketing strategy for Depo-Provera in Brazil away from the "narrow-market upper-income women." By financing an advertising campaign targeting "key government" actors and "professional associations," and consolidating "strategic partnerships" between the private and public sectors (22), the Futures Group, with funding from USAID, helped Pharmacia-Upjohn exceed its sales projections by 30 percent, primarily among the low-income bracket of the Brazilian population. In Bahia, the escalation in the distribution of hormonal injections in public health sector services is evident in the official figures I obtained from the state of Bahia's Health Division.[7] According to these figures, the number of trimonthly hormonal injections distributed by the state of Bahia alone (that is, excluding those bought directly over the counter) increased spectacularly from 354 units in 1994 to 45,675 in 2003. Although no comparable statewide data are available for subsequent periods because the data-collecting service was discontinued, in 2008 health providers in three distinct family planning centers in Salvador estimated that Depo-Provera, or its "copy," Contracep, accounted for more than half of the contraceptive methods they had distributed the previous month.[8] Alongside this method, second-generation oral contraceptive pills figure prominently in state-funded services. There is seldom any choice in the type of pills available at any one time (although women often state a preference for one type), and it is common for stocks to vary from one month to the next, such that women may not always find the pill they were previously administered in their local health dispensary. Public ambulatórios generally administer pills by packs of three, and pill users often return to find that the pill they have been using is no longer available. This renders whatever else is available interchangeable, by default, inverting the logic of choice into a logic of necessity, of sorts. In these public services, teenage girls are often proposed the injection in place of the pill, when it is available. One doctor I interviewed justified this as follows: "The injectable is much more effective. . . . That way, we know for sure the patient won't get pregnant and that we are not wasting resources." Injectable contraceptives are pitched as a reliable alternative to the pill for young women who are presented as esquecidas (forgetful). In Salvador, much attention is given to the risky sexual practices of teenage girls leading to unwanted pregnancy (see Marinho, Aquino, and Conceição 2009). The discrepancy between national guidelines concerning contraceptive choice provision and the reality on the ground is in part the result of an incomplete process of devolution of the responsibility for family planning service provision from the Ministry of Health in Brasília to state- and municipal-level services. These various factors and the organizational challenges of providing a homogeneous service in a country marked by profound regional differences contribute to substantially constraining choice locally. In private-sector consultations, emphasis is placed on individualized choice (seeped in a consumer, rather than a rights-based, logic) or on the personalization of services—even when this is merely symbolic or discursive. By contrast, as I show in the following section, the administration of hormonal contraceptives and the treatment of persons in public services are carried out in a highly depersonalized and "massified" manner.

Disciplining the Population, Regulating the Body of the Nation

The distribution of contraceptive methods in the state of Bahia was administered through an information technologies system called SISPF until the mid-2000s. This system effectively traded contraceptive methods for data (e.g., the number of new and returning patients, demographic data about which methods were distributed); municipalities were requested to send in data about contraceptive methods distributed to ensure their continued supply.[9] Calculations of the contraceptive target were elaborated on the basis of existent demand and the annual contraceptive goal. This percentage was computed from estimates of the population of nonsterilized women of fertile age and of women dependent on the SUS, which generated a figure for the contraceptive demand, that is, the annual number of women for whom contraception needed to be provided. SISPF was set up to address a specific concern with the problem of "choice" of contraceptive methods, ensuring that the distribution of future methods would be indexed on existent demand (which varies from one municipality to the next). Demand thus became a means of fixing goals. SISPF was unique to Bahia and was elaborated on the initiative of CRESAR, an organ of the *Secretaria de Saúde* State Department of Health that grew in autonomy throughout the 1990s and was initially supplied in contraceptives by Pathfinder and USAID. Under recent SUS reforms, family planning has been devolved to the system of "basic health units," and CRESAR—whom North American organizations had since stopped supplying—re-specialized in training and monitoring family planning activities. The reshuffling in the administration of reproductive health in Salvador, and Brazil more generally, seeks to integrate this into other basic medical services dispensed through the SUS. The problem is that in "basic health" provision, targets are set in response to specific health concerns that require the prioritization of certain health actions over others. Here, epidemiological data on health priorities confront institutional constraints regarding the provision of solutions to these, in conjunction with—or at the expense of—other aspects of the integrated health agenda.

With regard to family planning, the epidemiological focus that informs public health prioritizations reveals a drop in fertility, which has led certain aspects of "sexual and reproductive health" to be prioritized over others. In a context where the idea that the national fertility rates need to be controlled continues to be widely rehearsed, the provision of family planning services has paradoxically declined as contraceptive methods fail to reach dispensaries and reproductive health is not yet fully set in motion in many basic health units.[10] In a series of meetings with Murillo, the *Secretaria's* IT coordinator who was responsible for the elaboration and running of health statistic programs, I was invited to consider the issue from the perspective of the generation of data about the population. As Murillo explains, there are conflicting interests at play at the level of the administration of health services that reveal the way the population is both imagined and constituted as a site of intervention. Murillo feels that the viability of SISPF has been directly challenged by the introduction of SISPrenatal, a system introduced by the (federal) Ministry of Health. SISPrenatal is a tool developed by DATASUS[11] to oversee the national program for the "Humanization of Prenatal Care and Birth."[12] This is a "paying system," as each *gestante* (pregnant woman) recruited before her fourth month of pregnancy generates income (R$10) for the health unit. A further R$40 is generated if she completes six prenatal consultations, and a hospital delivery generates R$40. Given that the same units are responsible for both prenatal care and family planning, and that family planning generates no income, health provision units are prioritizing prenatal care over family planning services. In other words, there is a direct conflict of interest between these two systems. The unintended consequence of the introduction of SISPrenatal has been a reduction in family planning services, as "*gestantes* bring in money, whilst family planning clients only cost," Murillo concluded.

This was translated in the ambulatórios by the distinction made between good and bad patients, and by the emphasis that staff placed on women adequately following the protocols. Those who do are "good patients" and congratulated. Those who do not are shunned and seen to impede the process and development of an adequate and functional system. It was common to hear staff tell women off for taking up space, using up scarce resources, or having a responsibility toward health providers who were struggling to make the system work. Here the logic of patient rights becomes one of patient responsibilities. When I was invited to consider the fact that complying with the prenatal protocol generated income for a unit, these disciplinary strategies became more intelligible to me, as did the comparative (and somewhat puzzling) laxness of family planning service provision. Many of the micro-interactions I observed in public-sector or nongovernmental family planning services are directed at getting women to "take responsibility," in a context where birth control is seen as integral to lifting the nation out of underdevelopment. In this neo-Malthusian vision, poverty is considered to be the result of excessive fertility, rather than its cause. Here, taking responsibility is part of constructing oneself as a (good) citizen. Good patients are those who comply with medical protocols and display proficiency with regard to both medical and institutional protocols. The terms cidadania (citizenship) and direitos (rights) are often invoked to discipline patients into fulfilling their obligations as good citizens, as illustrated in the following exchange between a gynecologist and his patient during a family planning consultation in a SUS maternity unit.

Doctor: Good morning, lindinha (pretty), when did you menstruate?
Patient: I think it was ... well, it finished about ... a few days ago.
Doctor: When did your menstruation start?
Patient: I don't remember the exact date, but it finished maybe a week ago ...
Doctor: It's not when it finishes that matters, it's when it starts.
Patient: I don't remember ...
Doctor (annoyed): Ah filha (daughter)! You have to know these things. Não é só tudo direito aqui (It's not just all "rights" here), you also have responsibilities. You have to responsabilizar-se (take responsibility) not to get pregnant.
Patient: I think it was on the eleventh?

Joking was often used to convey not-so-subtle messages concerning reproductive behavior in these contexts.[13] Many doctors feel disheartened by the degree of ignorancia (ignorance) they see themselves as being confronted by in their work in SUS ambulatórios. Despite their continued efforts to provide family planning information and services, "cultural beliefs" are seen to impede the appropriate use of contraceptive methods. Public health clinical encounters have a double agenda in that, through them, actions on the population are sought. At the level of the clinic, they are often concerned with the production of "good patients," and much of the — extremely short — consultations are directed at treating ignorancia. On one occasion, a receptionist interrupted a consultation I was observing to tell the doctor that a woman had been admitted explaining that she was perdendo (losing [the baby/blood]). The doctor looked up and retorted: "Well help her find it then!," to which they both laughed. Similarly, sterilization is often referred to as ligar (which literally means "to tie" or "to make a phone call"). Semantically, this implies that what is tied can be untied, a "myth" that doctors at times attempt to dispel, while at times using the term themselves.[14] For example, after beating around the bush during a morning outpatient clinic, a woman finally asks: "Tell me doctor, could I ligar?" Joking, the doctor picks up the phone, hands it to her and says, "Sure, just tell me the number!" She looks as surprised as I am, but he continues: "It's not a ligação [call/tie], it's a permanent sterilization." She insists and asks if they "go through the belly-button" or "make a cut," explaining that she would prefer a keyhole surgery, because her cesarean scar is tão bonita (so pretty) and she does not want to ruin it. She is knowledgeable about the different protocols and her institutional dexterity and manner soften the initially irritated doctor. She acquires information about how to obtain the procedure despite the fact that she has only two children at thirty-four. When she leaves — with a prescription for the trimonthly hormonal injection — I ask the doctor why he did not suggest that her partner come for a vasectomy (given that she has told us that he has five children), but he shrugs this off, explaining that "machismo" prevents Bahian men from considering the option. Plus, he adds, she is decided, and she will get her surgery no matter what he advises. This example reveals the ways in which the relative display of knowledge or ignorancia in turn facilitates a more or less personalized atendimento on behalf of health professionals.

Women have various strategies to deal with mistreatment from medical staff. Some of these include withholding, or giving minimal, information. During a focus group I ran on menstruation and contraceptive use with women from a favela, I asked one young woman about her preferred method. She assertively retorted that she was a virgin and, mocking me, recounted an experience with a gynecologist who had assumed — as I had — that she was sexually active and had asked her questions about her sexual activity. In her narration it became clear that she had not revealed his error to the doctor and allowed him to continue, mechanically, his line of inquiry. She was prescribed a *preventivo* (Pap test) and a transvaginal ultrasound, she added, raising her eyebrows in defiant amusement. I asked whether she had told the doctor she preferred a transabdominal one, but she replied: "*Pra que, né?! Peguei um ignorante* [What for, hey?! I landed on an ignorant one]. I limited myself to responding to his questions." Conversation immediately flowed on patient–doctor miscommunication, revealing that this group of young women was astutely aware of the ways doctors try to catch them out and test their knowledge about contraceptive use. Withholding information, or imparting partial and, at times, deliberately erroneous information, is a means of carving out a space of autonomy in the restrictive space of ambulatório protocols. Women spoke more readily to friends and kin to elaborate strategies for themselves, based on their common embodied experiences, rather than comply with the disciplining of the national body that family planning—in its emphasis on population—effectively promotes (see de Zordo 2012). Similarly, Gonçalves et al. (2011, 210) found that young women at times mobilized the stereotype of the reproductively prolific lower-class woman in jest, as a way of resisting inappropriate but widely held conceptualizations of the poor. Asked whether her pregnancy had been planned, Susana, a young woman they introduce, responded off-hand, "poor people don't plan pregnancies, now, do they?!"

Humor at times served to spell out responsibilities, making hierarchies and gendered norms at times painfully obvious. For example, in a maternity unit where family planning services were dispensed in the context of postnatal revisions, a woman entered with her newborn for a postpartum revision and the doctor asks, "Everything all right?" "Only a headache, doctor," she answers, to which he responds, "That's the *juízo* [judgment] arriving to take care of the baby." The woman nods passively and says, "Doctor, I wanted to schedule my surgery," and he responds, "What surgery, *querida* [darling]?" "I want to *ligar* [tie/sterilize], doctor." "But you are only twenty-seven," he replies, looking at the form in front of him. She tells him this is her sixth child. "Well then it really was lack of *juízo* and we're going to intern you in a monastery!" he jokes. Half-amused, she responds that she doesn't want to, and he replies, "Then your problem is a problem of faith *querida*, and I can't help you!" The patient leaves with a prescription for the trimesterly injectable contraceptive that is often given to nursing mothers. On the same morning, a woman of thirty-one comes in for her postpartum revision. She is missing teeth and her clothes are ragged. The doctor asks if the birth was *cesaria* (cesarean delivery) or *normal* (vaginal), and she answers that it was a cesaria, reminding him that he had scheduled it in order to perform a tubal ligation at the same time. "How many children?" the doctor asks, looking up from the form for the first time. "Eight," the woman answers. "Oh, I remember," the doctor says. "Your husband wanted to make a football team, and he was even going to make the other side and the referee, but we stopped him!"

The first tubal ligation that I attended was performed on a woman of twenty-six who had had eight pregnancies and borne six children.[15] When I entered the operating theater with the doctor, she was lying naked—her dark body marked by poverty—on the operating table, waiting for the anesthetic. The head nurse, a strict black matron, announced to the doctor: "This one here is only twenty-six and already has eight. Can you imagine something like this today, with all the possibilities of planning! *Não existe!* [this doesn't exist!]."

The woman does not say a word as the staff vigorously scrub her down with a yellow disinfectant and the doctor noisily slips on his rubber gloves. CEPARH, where I was allowed to observe a range of surgical procedures, was greatly appreciated by low-income patients because it is a private clinic that offers charitable treatment free of charge. Here, sterilizations are performed using keyhole surgeries rather than full abdominal incisions. Although the nonpaying patients attended to "downstairs" are treated very differently from the paying patients attended to "upstairs" (the two services even have distinct entrances on different roads), they often expressed appreciation for the more personalized treatment they received at CEPARH, exemplified through such things as the keyhole surgery, the tone of the reception staff, or simply the access to a famous, private clinic. These cases demonstrate how stigmatizing ignorance and noncompliance with protocols can be, and how the display of knowledge and the negotiation of access to services can be mobilized by patients as a form of capital. As we shall see, this needs to be understood in the Brazilian context within the frame of the highly specific meanings that notions such as "rights" and "responsibilities" take on. In the remainder of this section I turn to the clearance interviews that vasectomy "candidates" undergo to reveal the ways in which these enjoinders to take responsibility are negotiated differently according to gender, race, and class distinctions.

At CEPARH, all family planning patients have an interview with a social worker, as part of a protocol laid out by World Health Organization recommendations. In the case of male and female sterilization, the goal is to evaluate the person's familial situation and determination to have the procedure, in order to avoid *arependimento* (regret).[16] CEPARH actively promotes vasectomy over female sterilization, and during the course of fieldwork I witnessed over fifty social service consultations with "vasectomy candidates" and a dozen vasectomy surgeries. The formal criteria used to evaluate vasectomy "candidates" include the number of children a couple have together, the duration of their relationship, their respective ages, and the ages of their children. In practice, however, patients are *liberado* (approved) on what seem to be highly subjective grounds.[17] Race and class are implicitly salient in the decision process to approve a man for vasectomy. Because CEPARH's ambulatório is one of the few places that provides vasectomies free of charge in Salvador, the range in socioeconomic background of vasectomy candidates varies much more than it does for women, among whom the concentration of low-income patients is considerably higher. CEPARH, as we have seen, is fairly unique in that the free, philanthropic (public) or the high-quality (private) dimensions can be mobilized by both patients and staff at different moments. The social worker is acutely aware of this and particularly attentive to her *meninos* (boys), attending to them first, and with longer, friendlier consultations, in order to "'*incentivize*' men to *responsibilizar-se* [take responsibility for themselves]," as she explains.

One morning, a forty-five-year-old, white, middle-class man enters Dona Maria's office, in answer to her call: "number 3!" Somewhat ironically, while doctors call patients by their names, the social worker calls them by the number they are given in order of arrival. He is clearly uncomfortable after the wait in the noisy, non-air-conditioned waiting area, cramped with women from the *periferia* (low-income suburbs). As the conversation unfolds, he explains his recent loss of employment (and private health insurance), negotiating his (equal) position in relation to the social worker. She is surprisingly warm, and the consultation begins with a discussion that establishes that they have common acquaintances, further confirming a social equilibrium in what is usually a very hierarchical situation. The man explains that he has four sons ranging from thirty years to five months of age. His two eldest, and the wife and children of the eldest, live with his ex-wife, for whom he provides. The second two children he had with his current wife, with whom he had difficulty conceiving their first child. Given these difficulties, after this birth the couple did not use any contraception, and the newborn came as a complete surprise, at a difficult economic time. He presents his choice to undergo vasectomy as "taking care of her" and taking "responsibility" for his existing children and grandchildren. Dona Maria is touched by the story; the tone of the encounter is very different, given the social proximity that has been established between the patient and social worker. Normally, vasectomy candidates are not approved if their youngest child is under the age of one because the risk of losing the child is considered to be high until this age is reached. In this context, the objective criteria defined by national guidelines for good practice (the number of children in the current relationship and age of the last born) would normally have led to a refusal of the patient. When he leaves, she turns to me, enchanted, and exclaims: "What a good man! If they were all like this our country would be uma maravilha [wonderful]."

"Number 5!" is more representative of the population attended to by CEPARH's ground-floor ambulatório. He is a thirty-three-year-old black man and father to two children. He works in a borracharia (garage) and is married to Monica, twenty-one, the mother to his two declared children. They live in her mother's house (eight inhabitants for two rooms). He is humbly dressed, quiet and withdrawn in his responses, such as when he explains that he has not completed primary school education. He sticks firmly, but monosyllabically, to his position. When she sees the birth certificates of the children and Monica's identity card, Dona Maria comments in a mocking, friendly reprimand: "Monica is only a girl! She had children very early, didn't she? You took her right from the cradle, didn't you, danado [naughty]?" He plays along, slightly uneasy and unsure, attempting to gain her sympathy to his cause. "Porque que o senhor não quer mais filhos?" (Why does the gentleman not want any more children?), she asks in a monotone, mechanical voice. "Because, I think a casal [a boy and a girl] is sufficient, né?," the man responds, taken off guard. This response is normally deemed totally insufficient, and at times reprimanded. When on the previous day a young, well-dressed salesman had responded that he thought his casal was sufficient, she had interjected, "Think? You have to actually know!" Today she does not pick up on the response and begins to explain the procedure to him, indicating that he has been liberado (approved). I ask her why she has approved him, given the objective criteria that would speak against his case. She answers that he had a decided, affirmative attitude, which is quite debatable given the exchange.

The following week we meet a young black man of twenty-seven, married to a woman of twenty-four and father to four children by three different mothers. He is an unemployed builder and she is an unemployed domestic employee. "Has not completed basic education," Dona Maria spells out almost jovially as she writes down his hushed response to her question. She asks for the ages of the children and he answers that the first two are five. "Twins!" she exclaims enthusiastically, but he explains that they are by two different mothers. "Já pensou!" (Can you imagine!), she says, turning to me, in a joking, I've-seen-everything-now manner. The third is the second-born of one of the two mothers, and the fourth (aged two) is his current mulher (woman's) only child. Looking at the children's birth certificates, Dona Maria notes that the first two are born on the same day: November 17. "Did you just register them both that day?," she asks, unimpressed. He explains that they were born on the same day, to two women, and that he went to visit both mothers on that day. "Well, there's no doubt that they are not twins then," she jokes, amused again.[18] "Are you sure that you don't want any more children?," she asks mechanically. "Certain," he responds. "I shouldn't liberar you," she continues. "Your wife is young and only has one child. You are young too but you already have four, it's her who is going to remain with only one child. Are you sure?" He nods, decidedly, and is approved, with the thump of her stamp on his form. "Seguinte! [Next!], number 8!" She shouts out the open door.

These materials, collected through observations of vasectomy triage, are presented in detail because they provide an interesting contrast to the observations of family planning consultations addressed to women. What I wish to highlight through these examples is the way in which the personalization of atendimento is negotiated in this ambivalent space between private and public health care. The racial, class, and gendered dynamics that underscore these encounters give a highly subjective orientation to the way norms and guidelines are interpreted and negotiated. There is more room for negotiation here than there is for women negotiating access to sterilization, around which there is a degree of taboo, although it is still widely practiced.[19] CEPARH is proud of its vasectomy service, which is presented as a forward-looking approach to family planning through its inclusion of men in reproductive health care.

Hormonal Enhancement and Strategies of Self-Control

Things look very different in the parallel system of private health. One can trace similar contraceptive protocols and indeed pharmaceuticals across both sectors, but while in public family planning services the emphasis is on population control, here the rationale accompanying the administration of hormonal regimes is one of self-control. Subdermal hormonal implants tend to get classified with injectable contraceptives as methods that target the global poor in efforts to curtail fertility (e.g., Mintzes et al. 1993). In Brazil, however, the marketing and price of hormonal implants have produced these methods as consultório [private practice] treatments, that is, as elite consumer products that were only made available to low-income women during clinical trials.[20] Hormonal implants are marketed through extensive media coverage to middle-class women as drugs for the modern lifestyle— particularly with reference to the fact they are said to free a woman from menstruation. For example, Nova's (Cosmpolitan Brasil) February 2009 issue contained a feature in the "Health" section entitled "Beach—Menstruation free" (Na praia sem menstruar), outlining how to "free your white shorts and your bikini from the red deluge," thanks to hormonal implants. The emphasis is on remapping the possibilities of the body, and on a particular kind of sexual optimization. In addition to Organon's single-rod Implanon, a variety of hormonal implants are available in Salvador, as we shall see in detail in chapter 5. CEPARH produced its own implants from a variety of steroid sex hormones. These implants combine various hormones in "individualized" doses said to match the patient's profile. Testosterone is often added (either as additional capsules or prescribed as a transdermal gel) to boost sexual desire. Beatriz, a businesswoman I interviewed who has used hormonal implants for five years, described its effects in the following manner: "Hormônio acts in the brain. It gives a sensation of well-being, of disposition, it acts on muscles, it tones. It also interacts with the emotional part, and gives you control over those ups and downs. You feel prettier, sexier, everything, hair, skin, body, libido, muscle tone responds more quickly to stimulation. . . . So why live without libido? Without disposition for life? I'm totally in favor of hormônio."

In this sense, taking responsibility operates in a much less explicit—if equally pervasive—manner among middle-class women. In Salvador, when a man has an extramarital affair, it is not uncommon to hear it said that it is his wife's fault for failing to look after herself or maintain the tesão (sexual desire) in the relationship. The range of esthetic procedures women are tacitly expected to adopt in order to achieve these goals is ever expanding and includes weekly visits to the beauty parlor, cosmetic surgery, a constant monitoring of weight, attention to dress, hair, skin, and so on. Mood, being bem humorada (good-humored) or "disposed" (sexually but also, more generally, socially), is also key, as we have seen in previous chapters, and sex hormones are given a central role in modulating affects.

Late one evening, at a social gathering in an opulent flat filled with contemporary art overlooking the Bay of All Saints, a conversation spontaneously began between a group of women in their mid-forties concerning the hormones they were using. Alícia, our host, explained she had had trouble renewing her implants after her cardiologist noticed an increase in her cholesterol levels. After some negotiation she managed to obtain new implants and was impressed with how rapidly she had recuperated her sexual disposition and what she called her "quality of life." I asked her about her cholesterol, but she brushed off the risks, stating that the advantages far outweighed any concerns she could have. It struck me that the stakes of maintaining a particular social standing, which often implies—for women like her—securing their marriage, were a peculiar exercise in risk management. Alícia uses the implant as a form of contraception, but what emerges from the account she gives of her choice is the importance of its extracontraceptive properties: in this case the prestige associated—in Salvador—with this expensive method and the sexual enhancement she feels it confers.[21] A common friend explained to me a few days later on our way to explore what yoga hormonal therapy classes had to offer that Alícia's husband is "the one with the money" and that he is a notorious womanizer, often sleeping with girls barely older than their son. This, my friend implied, explains why keeping up libido, *disposição* (disposition), and appearances—through plastic surgery, dieting, elaborate workout regimes, and shopping in São Paulo's most exclusive boutiques—is so critical for Alícia.

The pill has been widely heralded as making possible the severance between reproduction and sexuality. The freedom purportedly conferred to women by this separation of sexuality from reproduction has nevertheless been questioned. Though it broke away with earlier moral attitudes toward sex (as legitimate only in the context of reproduction), the budding field of sexology research saw in the increase of women's orgasmic potential a key to promoting marital stability.[22] In his cultural history of testosterone, Hoberman (2005, 7) notes that estrogen therapies were widely adopted in the postwar era as a means of promoting efficiency among the female workforce and providing husbands with "more satisfying sexual partners." This leads him to speak of a form of "drug-induced sexual fitness" that can be experienced "as a mandate to be sexually active even in the absence of desire" (8).

Cleonice is in her mid-forties and married to an architect from the south of Brazil. I met her at CEPARH, where she was having her implants renewed, and she agreed to an interview. She has been using implants for over a decade. She describes herself as *mestiça* and has had several "minor" (in her words) *plásticas* (to the eyelids, nose, and facelift). "*Gosto de me cuidar* [I like caring for myself]," she explains, "and hormones help me feel good, they help the body, the skin. It improves your *performance* [in English], you have more *disposition*." Asked what she means by "disposition," Cleonice emphasizes first that hormônio gives her "energy to face her day-to-day, with more *vontade* [will]." Although the doctors I observed prescribing implants usually referred to testosterone as *dar fogo* (to give fire, an explicitly sexual metaphor), patients tended to emphasize wider dispositional changes. Asked about whether hormones affect sexual desire as well, Cleonice responds: "It does a lot of good, it brings tremendous well-being, not just physical, but mental and emotional too. I think it really helps. The doctor says adding testosterone will give *fogo*, and I think the term is very appropriate. It literally does give you fogo! [laughs]." Cleonice, like many women I encountered, spoke explicitly of hormônio and her plásticas in terms of cuidar-se: "It's very important for people to *cuidar da aparência* [care for appearance], to care for esthetics, to be in good sexual and emotional disposition, to keep the body in shape through exercise and diet and to fix what needs fixing."

The "disposition" procured by hormones is often set against the emotional and physical discomforts associated with regular menstruation, in particular with so-called premenstrual tension, as we saw in previous chapters. Menstrual suppression using Mirena, hormonal implants, or oral contraceptives is widely presented as a means of regulating emotions associated with menstruation, such as irritability, sadness, anger, or sluggishness. As far as the presentation of these hormonal regimes is concerned (in the media or during private-sector consultations), the contraceptive properties come to be almost secondary to the lifestyle aspects of the drug that are put forward. I found that private-sector patients are often encouraged in medical consultations to consider sex hormones in terms of the affective changes they make possible, or in relation to such extracontraceptive properties. By contrast, when during consultations low-income women raise concerns with the side effects of the hormonal methods they are administered, these are often dismissed. Weight gain, headaches, and discomfort are common complaints among pill and injection users in public health services. Medical professionals sometimes brush off complaints as ignorance, stating that there is no connection between the use of hormones and such side effects, or that it is "in their [patient's] head." Weight gain is a substantial concern among all hormone users. Although the link between certain hormonal methods such as Depo-Provera or certain types of hormonal implants and pills and weight gain has been established, I often heard low-income patients be told: "Food causes weight gain, not hormones." Yet one of the most successful pills in Bahian private practices is a fourth-generation pill containing the hormone drospirenone (retailing under the brand name Yasmin, its national "similar" copy Dalyne, and several generic versions), widely lauded as the "weight loss" pill (see Sanabria 2014). Drospirenone's diuretic effects have been intensively scripted through advertising to signify *bem-estar* (well-being). Marketing emphasizes a "truly different" pill "shown repeatedly to have no associated weight gain" and to improve PMS symptoms. In Bahia, drospirenone is presented as *um aliado eficaz na redução dos sintomas da* TPM (an efficient ally in reducing PMT symptoms), according to a pamphlet found in a gynecologist's waiting room. It is above all known as *a pilula que emagrece* (the weight-loss pill), or the pill that reduces swelling. This claim is never sustained officially or in writing. But the regional pharmaceutical reps who promote Yasmin or its copies to gynecologists never failed to summarize the effects in this manner, well aware of the local importance of the trope of *inchaço* (swelling) in relation to hormônio.[23] So, while private-sector patients are invited and, indeed, encouraged to consider the effects of the hormonal regimes beyond their prescribed functions, the experiences of public-sector patients are not always taken seriously, highlighting once more the way differentiations are made between these two categories of users.

Sex Hormones: "Molar" and "Molecular" Biopolitics

Sex hormones operate regulatory control at several distinct levels (including the regulation of the reproductive functions of the body). As contraceptives, standardized drugs are distributed en masse in an effort to regulate the body politic through the bodies of the "poor," where hormonal regimes are involved in "treating" ignorance and underdevelopment. Expensive pharmacotechnologies developed to administer hormones (such as subdermal implants or intrauterine hormonal systems) are marketed to specific patient profiles, who are invited to make "individualized" choices to discipline subjectivities, enhance the self, and regulate affective flows. The apparently trivial question of pharmaceutical sex hormone packaging and administration reflects and reproduces social differences, such as those between sub- and super-citizens. The suggestion is that this distinction is replicated in the question of drug packaging and that these social distinctions can in turn be mapped onto an additional set of distinctions, such as between standardizing and individualizing treatments of persons, or between a focus on the population (concern with demography) and a focus on the individual (concern with subjectivity). In this sense, I argue that the administration of pharmaceutical sex hormones in Brazil reveals a differentiating form of citizenship that can be mapped onto the two forms of biopolitics enunciated by Foucault (1976, 183) and elaborated on by Rabinow (1996) and Rose (2007).

In the remainder of the chapter I address the coexistence of differences in health care provision within the Brazilian polity from the perspective of debates on the governing of bodies. Current developments in the life sciences have brought about a renewed interest in Foucault's notion of "biopolitics" (e.g., Novas and Rose 2005; Rabinow 1996; Rose 2007). Rabinow (1996, 91) has argued that the two poles of biopower identified by Foucault—"the anatomo-politics of the human body" and "the regulatory pole centered on the population"—are being rearticulated into what he called "a post-disciplinary rationality." Rose (2007) argues for a historical transition from the biopolitics of the population that marked the nineteenth and twentieth centuries to that of the "self," which, in his view, characterizes the twenty-first century. In the contemporary mode, "corporeal existence"—no longer understood as fate, but actively modulated and increasingly molecularized—has become "the privileged site of experiments with the self" (26). Rabinow and Rose (2006) adopt the distinction between "molar" and "molecular" modes of power to differentiate between actions led at the level of populations and collectivities from what they call the "individualization of biopolitical strategies." Interestingly, Rose (2007, 11) later classifies hormones—along with blood, tissues, organs, and limbs—on the "molar" side of the equation, effectively attributing them to the "old" clinical medicine with its focus on the "the visible, tangible body." This dichotomy is essentially set up to reveal something of the novelty of molecular genomics (the new "molecular" pole of biopower). My suggestion is that sex hormones are interesting precisely because they operate at the boundary between these two biopolitical poles.

According to Rose, the new vital politics is led by biological citizens whose activism draws on novel biosocial identities or through the activities of individuals who modulate, adjust, and improve themselves by adopting technologies of "optimization." This renders the disciplinary dimension of these new practices of self-making rather opaque. In what follows I outline the way both the "old" and "new," or "molar" and "molecular," models of biopolitics are at work in Brazilian reproductive health practices, but argue that these are addressed to different segments of the Brazilian polity. The use made of sex hormones among many Bahian women resembles what Rose terms a new "neurochemical citizenship" in that these molecules are popularly understood as integral to mood, disposição, and sexual desire and adopted in strategies of self-making. However, although these hormonal praxes are geared toward forms of what we might call sexual and subjective "optimizations," they do not exist in a relational vacuum, as implied by Rose's notion of self-responsibility. Further, I question the extent to which we might characterize these activities of self-making as part of what he calls a "moral economy of hope." For Rose (2007, 148), hope—in the contemporary regime of biological truth—actively transforms the future, rather than merely anticipating it. However, the transformative potential of "hope" operates, for Rose, through active forms of democratic participation, which in Brazil remain constrained as far as biological citizenships are concerned. In what follows I examine some of the specificities of Brazilian health inequalities with reference to broader modes of differentiation between types of citizens. I then turn to locally defined questions of participation in health care, outlining the differences between these and the notion of active democratic participation that is central to Rose's notion of "hope."

Negotiating Impersonal Universals and Legalized Exceptions

As we have seen, technical and biomedical interventions on middle-class bodies have *personalizing* tendencies, whereas those effected on the bodies of the urban poor can be read as modes of inclusion through *standardization*. Much of Brazilian sociality can be read through this differentiation between standardized and personalized. In this section I show how the consumption of drugs and medical services is marked by this distinction. The public health system is widely held to be "impersonal," whereas private health capitalizes on the notions of individualizing and personalizing health care. Against these lines of differentiation, observed during fieldwork across the public and private health sectors in Salvador, is another line of differentiation that authors such as Biehl mark. Biehl (2005) poignantly recounts the lives of those who fall outside the remit of SUS triage and projects aimed at democratizing and "humanizing" medical care. He calls these persons "ex-human" in reference to the way marginalized people in Brazil come to fall outside the bounds of the law, that is, outside of the institutions that recognize humanness and confer rights. Building from the more extreme question of which lives are worth living (Biehl 2005, 22), I consider how social differentiations are re-embedded in biomedicine in Brazil. In my research at various intersections between the SUS and private health institutions, distinctions in treatment—both literal and symbolic—served to differentiate between "common citizens" and "private individuals."

This is one way in which we can read the way medically assisted childbirth in Brazil ranges unevenly from an absence of care and anesthetic in public maternity units to an epidemic of surgical births in private maternity wards. McCallum and dos Reis (2008) show that, in Salvador, women in public health maternity units give birth vaginally using low-tech procedures (which often include the artificial induction of labor without any analgesia). While the rate of cesarean births in public maternity units ranges between 10 and 30 percent, in the private sector it varies between 80 and 100 percent (41). "Normal" birth, as it is referred to locally, thus comes to be abnormal in private medical institutions. In her work on in vitro fertilization in Ecuador, Roberts (2008, 91) argues that Ecuadorian elites readily constitute their bodies as unprepared for normal pregnancy, which they associate with peasant or indigenous women, whose bodies are symbolically constituted as closer to nature. Roberts argues that in dissociating themselves from the category of the "normal" (lo normal), her informants constitute themselves as "reproductively modern" (93). This speaks to the ways in which, in Latin America, normality is associated with nature and modernity implies a move out of nature, which naturalizes intervention. In Brazil, to be urban and modern implies embracing various interventions, and although access to biomedical technologies or pharmaceutical regimes is unequal, the pace set by private sector consumption patterns institutes desires that span across the class spectrum. In this sense, biomedical operations and technologies of enhancement are deeply embroiled in class hierarchies. Roberts's point speaks more generally to one of the central questions I address here, drawing on DaMatta's distinction between sub- and super-citizens. DaMatta argues that Brazilian modernity operates on a central tension between a formal embracing of the principles of equality and individualism and a tacit hierarchical mode or relationality. To be somebody—rather than a mere cidadão (citizen)—involves circumventing laws or general rules. In this sense, Brazilian sociality introduces a separation between an "impersonal, universal law and a person who sees himself as special and deserving of personalized special treatment" (DaMatta 1991, 169). In practice, DaMatta (1991, 180) shows, this is played out as a tension between an emphasis on a universal law to be applied to all and the indignant response of the elites who demand a singular application of the law. In a famous essay entitled "Do You Know Who You Are Talking To?" DaMatta (1991) shows how Brazilians commonly use this phrase to reassert a difference in status and claim a hierarchically superior position in the face of equalizing situations or public encounters. He contrasts this to the use of the North American formula "Who do you think you are?!," which equalizes and counters claims to superiority. Placing oneself above cultural or legal norms—or differentiating oneself from lo normal—is thus central to being elevated out from the impersonal mass of individuals and acquiring what DaMatta calls "personhood," a sign of privilege in itself. This antinomy between the universalizing aspect of law applied to "common" citizens and the particularizing legalized exceptions of privilege finds a parallel in the logic of standardizing/personalizing pharmaceutical sex hormone administration examined here.

The case of abortion provides a particularly striking illustration of the legalized exceptions of privilege in Brazil (Alves et al. 2014; Aquino et al. 2012; Menezes and Aquino 2009; Menezes, Aquino and Oliveira da Silva 2006). Abortion, as we saw, is illegal, and low-income women, for whom the cost of a safe abortion in a private clinic is prohibitive, rely on a range of alternative techniques to induce abortion themselves. If complications ensue—as they often do—a woman will present herself to a public maternity unit, stating that she is having a spontaneous abortion. In Brazil, medical councils, police, and health authorities all know about the private clinics but generally turn a blind eye. In April 2008 a case hit the Brazilian news: a private clinic practicing abortion in Mato Grosso do Sul was brought to justice, and the files of nearly 10,000 women who had carried out abortions there were withheld by the police as evidence in the legal actions to be carried out against them. The female doctor who performed the abortions was imprisoned. The case stood out as exceptional, however. In these clinics, abortions are carried out by suction, under full anesthetic, such that the women do not engage with the aborted materials. Some authors (e.g., Leal and Lewgoy 1995) argue that low-income women explain abortion as menstrual regulation because they have a different "culture" (sic). Such analyses fail to account for the way in which these purported "cultural" differences are produced through the institutional contexts within which they unfold. These so-called cultural understandings of the body are as much the product of (modern) national regulations and legal frameworks surrounding reproduction as they are of "tradition" or "culture." As Menezes et al. (2006, 1444) note, most studies limit their focus to low-income groups without giving due consideration to the "unique Brazilian situation of extreme inequality" or to the heterogeneity of "family arrangements, and sociability networks" that shape practices of abortion.[24] This is another example of how, in Brazilian public health, the ideal of universal and equal treatment coexists with violent inequalities in the treatment of persons.

Bioavailabilities

Cohen (2005) borrows the pharmacological term *bioavailability* to examine the disaggregation of organs and tissues from living bodies and their transaction or reincorporation into other bodies. He traces the connections between bioavailability and operability, which is defined as the degree to which "belonging to and legitimate demands of the state are mediated through invasive medical commitment," such as surgical sterilization (86). I in turn borrow Cohen's notion of bioavailability, returning it to its primary pharmacological meaning, as the rate at which a drug enters the body and reaches its target organ or tissue. The question of bioavailability is at the heart of the differences in sex hormone packaging and administration that I have traced here. Nonoral hormonal methods were developed to circumvent first-pass metabolism,[25] which lowers the bioavailability of orally ingested drugs. The changes in dosage, modes of administration, or drug delivery mechanisms outlined here as changes in "packaging" aim to increase the bioavailability of sex hormones. While methods marketed to consultório patients discursively emphasize the close tailoring of treatments to natural hormonal levels or bodily states, those targeting the urban poor aim primarily at overcoming patient "misuse" and ensuring maximal contraceptive efficacy at a minimal cost. The (pharmacological) bioavailability of sex hormones is managed differently in the bodies of the urban poor than it is in those of the middle classes. Both groups are bioavailable, in the sense Cohen implies, but, as I have argued, hormonal contraceptives are made bioavailable in poor and elite women's bodies according to different logics. Key to this difference, I suggest, is the distinction that is made between "standardized" and "personalized." Teresa, a retired chemist and Spiritist, elaborated on the notion of personalizing medicinal treatments during an interview. She took hormone therapy for a number of years, despite—as she explains—a history of cancer (leukemia), following an exposure to benzene in her workplace.

> I took it [hormone replacement therapy] controlled, I did my exams, understand. But I didn't stop because of my propensity to develop cancer due to the modification of my blood from the exposure. No, the effect it gave in me was the disordered growth of my uterus due to the excessive quantity of hormônio. That's why they need more research on the pharmacology. Because the quantity that I need is not going to be the same as the quantity you need. So it was the dose that caused the problem, understand? . . . So I have a habit of saying "it wasn't the hormônio, it was the excess," the way it was administered. Because if I had the ideal quantity in my organism it would not have happened. . . . For me hormônio works very well, whether it is natural or artificial, the effect is the same. The only thing that I question is the dosage. Because we take it as a pill, one pill for everyone. And it is this excess that feeds the cancerous cells, that makes the uterus grow. Because every body is a body, everyone has their individuality. You will never find someone who is *igual* [equal/the same] to you.

As a chemist, Teresa is perhaps particularly able to articulate the relation between these questions of "dosage," as she refers to them, and the problem of standardization (a single pill for everyone) and personalization (the differences between bodies). This notion of personalization differs, I want to argue, from the notion of individualization that Rose (2007) and others place at the heart of the new regimes of biopolitics. In Salvador, the use of hormonal regimes among private-sector patients resonates with and differs from Rose's description of how individuals "are beginning to recode variations in moods, emotions, desires, and thoughts" (223) in molecular terms. Both the regulation of population and the modes of somatic individuality can thus be said to operate in Brazil, but the shift from one to the other can neither be spatialized nor historicized, as suggested. The coexistence of these different modes in Brazil has significant implications for locally defined issues of citizenship. As far as the services provided by the public health system are concerned, the population continues to have a very concrete existence in public health administration and to be disciplined, in keeping with the "old" model of biopower. In parallel, there exists a markedly different system of private health care in which sex hormones are deployed as part of strategies of self-optimization that Rose associates with the new mode of biopolitics. I now turn to the implications that Brazilian practices of private health care have for the "democratization" of the SUS and for the idea of health care as a universal, democratic right. In so doing I draw on a body of literature in Brazilian(ist) social theory that considers that the deep inequalities that mark Brazilian social life are reinforced by the coexistence of a system of citizenship founded on the notion of equality, and a system of patron–client relations that positions people hierarchically.

Democratization, Universalism, and Participation

Democratization has emerged as a key word in debates surrounding public health in Brazil. The term relates more generally to the vast process of political reform undertaken throughout the 1980s postmilitary transition and culminating in the constitutional reform of 1988, which stipulated, among other things, universal health care as a basic human right. Despite the creation of the SUS, with its emphasis on inclusion and universalism, the Brazilian population continues to be divided between those who have access to private health insurance and those who depend solely on the SUS.[26] My suggestion is that we can approach these processes of social differentiation anthropologically by considering how they are re-embedded in the relations formed within technoscientific practices. Holston (2008, 3–4) argues that although it is articulated in relation to the state, Brazilian citizenship "manages social differences by legalizing them in ways that legitimate and reproduce inequality." Like DaMatta (1987, 1991), Holston (2008) shows how in common usage, the term *cidadão* (citizen) is used to refer to someone of no significance—a nobody—and to indicate lack of influential relations. While elites benefit from privileges that place them above the law, and confer extra rights, for the common cidadão there is, as it were, nothing but the law. Current public debates concerning citizenship attempt to redress this institutionalization of inequality. For the most part, however, these efforts are directed at addressing the absence of fundamental rights (that is, of extending rights to those without them), but do not address the fact that members of the elite benefit from privileges that place them beyond the law.[27] Holston (2008, 5) argues that the Brazilian concept of citizenship "defines citizens as others.... Moreover, it considers that what such others deserve is the law—

not in the sense of law as rights but of law as disadvantage and humiliation, a sense perfectly expressed in the Brazilian maxim 'for friends, everything; for enemies, the law.'"

The "structural inferiors"—or sub-citizens—of the Brazilian system, referred to collectively as "the people" or "the poor," tend to be viewed by Brazilian elites (the super-citizens) as a "generalized" and "massified entity" (DaMatta 1991). Holston's work, in revealing the intricate ways in which the notion of civil rights is constructed in Brazil, reveals how, effectively, what is public and guaranteed in the law as a right is also understood as stigmatizing. What is more, the public—as configured through public policy—does not, in Brazil, explicitly include those attended to through the parallel private sector. For example, the (federal) state collects statistical data about the population attended to by the SUS. However, state-produced data on the "population" do not include data on private-sector patients. When, for example, I searched for information on the distribution of contraceptive methods among this group, I was referred to the sales figures held by pharmaceutical companies. This produces a distinction between how the two populations come to be known—through the state or through the market—as the state counts only the population it administers directly through the SUS, and there are no equivalent figures for the population attended to through private practices and clinics. How are we to think of this absence that effectively renders a whole section of the population beyond, or above, the domain of public policy? The implication this has for democratization in Brazil is that it continues to mark the emerging public domain—via the policy landscape—by a notable absence: that of the elites and middle classes who rely on private services.

In an article on the democratization of health, Martins et al. (2008) adopt a highly contextualized meaning for the notion of "participation," arguing that a significant portion of the population does not participate in public health. This results from what they refer to as the "exclusion" of the most well-remunerated layers of society "towards the private health system" (113). The idea of an "excluding universalization," initially proposed by Faveret and Oliveira (1989) barely a year after the SUS's inception, refers to the hybrid nature of Brazilian health care provision and to the absence of a significant portion of the population from public services. The "exit" of this group from public health has implications for health inequalities, reinforcing the idea that public services are merely services for the poor. This situation participates in the construction of "a society with two types of citizens" (Martins et al. 2008, 114). The concept of universality plays a pivotal role in Brazilian discourses on the consolidation of a democratic state of rights, such as the right to health. However, this ideal is at odds with the differentiated regimes of citizenship outlined above. In the course of fieldwork, I met Chico and Laurinha, the brother and sister-in-law of a close friend. Leading an alternative and politically engaged lifestyle with their three children, Chico and Laurinha had deliberately decided not to subscribe to any form of medical insurance. This was an exceptional choice in the middle-class context of which they nevertheless formed part. Chico, whose father had been a well-respected pediatrician in Salvador, explained to me that unless the middle classes started using the SUS and making demands on the public health service, things would never get better. As a white, educated, resourceful middle-class family, they certainly had the means to negotiate the complex bureaucracy and ensure correct treatment. I was often stuck by the differences in the way medical professionals treated people as a function of subtle class codes (such as physical appearance, propriety, cordiality, and knowledge of medical protocols). Educated, white patients occasionally did appear in public health dispensaries, but they tended to be treated much more courteously, and things denied to others were at times conceded to them as favors. In seeking to overcome the exclusionary inequality introduced by the coexistence of two health systems, Chico and Laurinha nevertheless benefit from the implicit accordance of privilege and favor—no doubt aided by Chico's network of connections, as the son of a well-respected doctor.

Although the terms *citizenship*, *responsibility*, and *rights*, among others, are common in Brazilian reproductive health services, they seldom operate in the way suggested by the figure of the active patient-citizen mobilized in Rabinow's or Rose's accounts of the new vital politics. Mendes (1996, 62–63), for example, notes that those who benefited from the creation of the SUS are not socially organized and do not have a political voice. He refers to them as the "silent majority" and notes that while they became medical citizens with the constitution of the SUS, they remain "political sub-citizens." For the urban poor, demarginalization and social inclusion often depend on choosing to be a responsible patient. The various regulatory strategies outlined above lead to questioning the extent to which we have entered what Rabinow (1996) has called a "post-disciplinary rationality." Although Rabinow notes that a complex imbrication of rationalities continues to exist, the accent in these approaches tends to be on the novel forms. Both Rabinow and Rose recognize the need for further empirical analyses of the biopolitical rationalities of the near future. However, the use of the pronoun *we* or of terms such as *self* and *the contemporary* (in the singular) runs the risk of overlooking the significant differences that exist even within contexts defined as "Western." My intention has been to outline how the distribution and access to biotechnological developments such as hormonal contraceptives or childbirth and abortion services in Brazil exacerbate social inequalities as different biopolitical rationalities coexist. There has been a welcome academic and policy focus on the exclusion of the most marginal from health services, but I wonder to what extent the SUS can be consolidated without greater recognition of another exclusion: that of the elites.

Contrasting ethnographic materials such as those presented here with recent debates on the biopolitical rationalities at play in the contemporary epoch allows interesting conceptual difficulties to emerge. A term such as *individual*, for example, carries — in the Brazilian context — different, impersonal connotations, being commonly set against that of *person* in ways that break with the kind of conceptual work that *individual* does in contexts such as those described by Rabinow (1996) or Rose (2007). Rabinow's is a rather horizontal notion of (bio)sociality. It worked to show how lay/expert lines of tension were undermined in contexts where patients became specific types of experts that challenged classic doctor–patient relationships. What this occults is the fracture lines in this horizontality, the places where the collective comes apart at the seams. In Brazil, elite modes of medical consumption often become a model for the popular classes: There is nothing accidental about the way press coverage of these technologies is managed. There is a powerful aspirational dimension to entering the biosocial that is not always realized, or that is perhaps doomed by capitalist logics to be always incomplete. The bio is always a becoming, not something that is given or foundational to identity in the sense that genetic or disease classifications are (Edmonds and Sanabria 2014). Perhaps one key manner through which we can move past the paradigm of biosociality is to take seriously the idea that biology and nature as categories occupy different places within local epistemologies and have different relationships to the social.

CHAPTER 5

SEX HORMONES

MAKING DRUGS, FORGING EFFICACIES

Historian Elizabeth Watkins (2012) argues that there is nothing innovative about the purportedly new hormonal methods currently available on the market. Their sole novelty, she argues, resides in the marketing of the secondary, or "lifestyle," effects of sex hormones. Watkins traces the tactics for "tinkering" with the pill's design, arguing that pharmaceutical companies promoted "distinctive aspects of what were essentially similar products" (1465). The introduction of slight variation supplants genuine innovation with mere imitation (1465). Interestingly, Watkins dwells less on the development of new modes of administration, concluding that the contraceptive options available to women today hardly differ from those available to their grandmothers (1464). This reveals the way Watkins constructs the notion of similarity. Her notion of "hardly different" hinges on the similarity of the active principles themselves. She shows the extent to which sex hormone marketing hinges on demonstrating differences within noncontraceptive properties of "new" products. However, her analysis runs the risk of overlooking the way in which, in practice, marketing produces *very different things*. Small innovations produce big differences for users and prescribers alike. There is perhaps nothing "new" to the levonorgestrel compounds used in Norplant implants, the Mirena intrauterine hormone-releasing "system," or emergency contraceptive Plan B. However, these are so different in the minds of the women, doctors, and pharmacists I interviewed that they do not even enter a common category.

Yolanda is a tall, enthusiastic woman in her late twenties. We met one day in the waiting room of a private clinic, where a gynecologist was running two hours late. She wears the characteristic smart office garb of pharmaceutical representatives, and has a black attaché case full, I imagine, of *amostras* (free samples). She is a pharmaceutical representative for Nuvaring, and is zealous about this "completely novel approach" to contraception. Nuvaring is a small silicone ring inserted in the vagina once a month. She explains to me that private practice doctors are keen on Nuvaring but that they have come up against taboos in prescribing this method. She pulls out of her attaché case a three-dimensional plastic model of the female reproductive organs, explaining that she gives one to each doctor so they can educate their patients about the vagina, showing them how and where to insert Nuvaring. "Although we live in a very sexualized culture here in Brazil," she explains, "women don't know their own anatomy and have very traditional ideas still." Organon-Brasil actively works on this sexual trope in its marketing strategies. Yolanda enthusiastically recounts an "event" she recently held in a sex shop for a group of female gynecologists. The objective, she explains, is for the gynecologist to become a purveyor of information about pleasure and sexuality and to have access to new ideas and information in this respect.[1] The doctors she "visits" feel that their patients are not "ready" for this new approach to contraception. As one female gynecologist I interviewed explained: "Nuvaring is such a lovely method. But women have all sorts of preconceptions about it. That they will lose it in their vagina, or that their husbands will feel it. You have to explain that the vagina is a closed cavity, that Nuvaring can't be felt, and then you still have to get them to overcome their hang-ups about putting their hand in their vagina."

In the process of expanding contraceptive choices to patients, Nuvaring arises as something radically different for caregivers. This dispenser mechanism may have been experimented with for over forty years and contain entirely uninnovative steroid compounds, but as it is taken up by users, this object arises as a markedly different thing. The logistics of its use (inserted for three weeks, removed, and then reinserted one week later) and the locale of application (the vagina) contribute to rendering the similar aspects (to the pill) almost negligible. Depending on the perspective adopted, this object arises either as just the same old thing in new garb (Watkins 2012) or as radically different. These differences may appear to end users so considerable as to lead them to lose sight altogether of the fact that they are using a hormonal contraceptive method. The logic of differentiating, through the multiplication of contraceptive options, is so powerful that women at times fail to associate new hormonal methods with their hormonal action. Many of the women who use the hormone-releasing Mirena intrauterine device or hormonal implants opt for these methods precisely because they do not like the pill. While hormonal injections remain closely associated with and interchangeable with the pill, Mirena and implants have come to be perceived, by users, as unrelated to the pill.

This brings me to reflect on the relationship between the form given to sex hormones, and to pharmaceuticals more generally, and their effects. I draw on this case to consider how form is linked to the status of objects, and to think through the relationship between form and materiality. The forms given to objects are closely related to their function, which, in the case of drugs, is to dissolve into bodies. What is interesting, in this case, is that difference is produced out of ostensibly similar things (see Hayden 2007, 2013 for an excellent discussion of the related question of drug copies). I suggest that these objects are imagined as a singularity as a result of their existence as pharmaceutical drugs. My concern here is with the politics of fact-building surrounding sex hormones and with the ideas that come to be embedded in these medical objects when they are manufactured into drugs. In the second half of the chapter I draw on the work of Tim Ingold, who examines the way the objectness of entities lies in the delimitation of their outward surfaces. Ingold (2010, 6) argues that surfaces are "interface[s] between the more or less solid substance of an object and the volatile medium that surrounds it. If the substance is dissolved or evaporates into the medium, then the surface disappears, and with it the object it once enveloped." Ingold's critique of material culture studies—which, he argues, takes objects for granted and occults the processes through which they come into being and dissolve—is, I argue, particularly useful for thinking about pharmaceuticals and their effects.

Historian Nelly Oudshoorn (1994) argues that the concept of sex hormones was stabilized because it was made into a class of drugs that could be marketed for a wide range of pathologies. But she is clear to note that the particular drug profiles that emerged from the manufacturing process were not self-evident. As I show here, as new contours are given to sex hormones, new efficacies (both social and embodied) are produced. I examine how these efficacies collapse analytic distinctions between "material" and "semiotic." Sex hormones are particularly propitious to processes of translation, given their history and the fact that, as pharmaceutical drugs, they were able to enter a range of cultural, political, and social domains. The production of sex hormones into drugs stabilized these complex, labile objects; that is, it gave substance and a particular efficacy to a set of statements. In this process the (social) uses and culturally defined benefits to be drawn from their side effects perpetually evolved and changed as they traveled. And, in facilitating this capacity to travel, the possibility for new forms to arise was provided. In what follows I explore the way in which differences in packaging, modes of administration, and drug presentation produce different effects in ways that are not just "symbolic."

These processes of repackaging sex hormones, like the "reformulation regimes" described by Pordié and Gaudillière (2014), lie at the interface between regulatory systems, innovation processes, and globally stratified pharmaceutical markets. From the outset, hormonal repackaging strategies capitalized on off-label uses.[2] Peterson (2014) proposes the notion of "chemical arbitrage" to account for the ways regional pharmaceutical market dynamics bear not only on prescription regimes and modes of administration but also on chemistry itself. Her work adds to an emerging body of literature on pharmaceuticals that looks beneath the drug package and examines the work that goes into producing drugs as bounded commodities and crafting their specific efficacies (see also Hayden 2007, 2013). Peterson's ethnography shows how pharmaceuticals move along extensive networks of wholesale active ingredients and drug traders that span licit and illicit institutions, often capitalizing on regional variations in how these distinctions are drawn. The distribution chains of global drug economies (from production to prescription and procurement) *inform* chemical materials such as pharmaceuticals, determining the uses to which they are put.[3] Drawing on Bensaude-Vincent and Stengers's history of chemistry, Peterson (2014) and Barry (2005) have developed the notion of pharmaceuticals as "informed materials." This points to the way that drugs are shaped in informational and material environments that become coconstitutive with their molecular properties. Pharmaceutical companies do not produce bare molecules, Barry (2005) notes. The molecules they produce are "part of a rich informational material environment, even before they are consumed" (59). Where hormones are concerned, this rich informational environment includes the labor of clinical trials as well as the marketing and media coverage for "new" treatments and their uses, the advice given by a friend or kin member, or the ontonorms (Mol 2013) that are inscribed in them during patient–provider interactions or discussions across the pharmacy counter.

The ethnographic materials presented here reveal how deeply enmeshed the various attributes of a drug's efficacy are. I focus on the interplay between the finished, bounded form given to the object and the tangible efficacies that modulations in form and active principles produce. Mode of administration, dosage, active principles, packaging, shape and color, branding, and the official or unofficial efficacies that circulate between marketers, prescribers, and users combine almost seamlessly. The various attributes of drugs' efficacies bleed into each other as discursive or semiotic elements become embedded in the thing itself, pervading the material efficacies afforded by specific active principles or modes of administration.

Crafting Hormonal Implants:
From Powdered Hormone to Social Efficacy

What is interesting about the mutation of primary into secondary effects (as discussed by Etkin 1992) or pharmaceutical repackaging practices is that they make evident the inherently fluid nature of pharmaceutical objects. The repackaging of these labile objects largely occurs behind closed doors, in factories where active principles are stockpiled, dosed, and pressed into pills or capsules to be packaged into blister packets (or where hormonal vaginal rings, intrauterine hormone-releasing systems, or hormonal implants are manufactured). In Brazil, however, this work of compounding active principles into branded pharmaceutical objects is not limited to the distant factories where pharmaceutical laboratories formulate and box their products. Within the Brazilian pharmaceutical landscape one finds a fairly unique genre of pharmacy known locally as *farmácias de manipulação* (compounding pharmacies), where pharmaceuticals are manufactured — or "manipulated" — on demand out of their constitutive active principles.

Farmácias de manipulação grew out of the pharmaceutical tradition as it existed prior to the advent of industrialized production and distribution of manufactured drugs, wherein chemists would make up formulas within a small laboratory at the back of the shop where these were sold. There has been a resurgence of these pharmacies, reinvented in the 1990s, in response to what is described by pharmacists in this sector as the excessive standardization of drugs. Farmácias de manipulação are found in every shopping center in Salvador, and there are about half a dozen national chains as well as numerous independent pharmacies. In 2009 the director of the Bahian Council of Pharmacists estimated that the sector held 10 percent of the pharmaceutical market in Brazil, and continues to expand. From the outside, farmácias de manipulação present as clinical environments, with glass shelves displaying a selected line of beauty products, herbal substances, or dietary supplements. Behind the counter, a window offers a view into a laboratory where technicians go about their business. At the counter, patrons present their prescription, which is entered into the system, generating a time for pickup. The aesthetic of these pharmacies tends to be directly opposite to that of the drugstore pharmacy, privileging uncluttered surfaces and natural iconography (leaves, flowers, clouds, etc.). A door to the side of the counter leads to a corridor that runs through to the semi-solids lab (where gels or creams are manipulated), liquids lab (for syrups, solutions, or suspensions), and solids lab (for capsules). According to the stringent regulation of these pharmacies, these must be clearly differentiated and sealed-off environments. Each laboratory usually comprises a vent, a workbench, and a series of cupboards in which the substances to be manipulated are stocked. Here vats of emblematically allopathic products such as cortisone or anti-inflammatory drugs are stocked alongside herbal and mineral substances. Compounded remedies commonly mix pharmaceutical compounds, minerals, herbs, and vitamins and can be produced into solid, semi-solid, or liquid preparations, depending on the purpose and mode of administration. A key selling point is that of "individualizing" medicines. The idea is that the standardized packaging of drugs makes little sense, given that each individual is unique and metabolizes substances differently. This tailoring to the patient's individuality is pitched against the standardized practices of the pharmaceutical industry, which produces drugs en masse, without differentiation. The extensive regulation of this process of object making is guided by the logic of guaranteeing the quality of the end product: the ensuing manipulated drug-object. But according to the pharmacists I interviewed who worked in farmácias de manipulação, this extensive regulation is also the outcome of Big Pharma's lobbying activities. Both Brazilian and foreign pharmaceutical corporations, I was told, actively campaign within national regulatory instances to impede the spread of farmácias de manipulação, which, in populating the already densely saturated Brazilian pharmaceutical landscape, are taking away an important share of their market. But beyond profit per se, what is at stake here is the relationship that these large corporations create between active principles and clearly bounded, carefully marketed products (or objects), whose names ultimately come to stand for their pharmacological components, and the disease entities that their appearance on the market promotes. The regulation of this activity also attests to the volatile qualities of these materials, particularly at the point at which they are manipulated out of jars, pots, and containers and into objects of various kinds (pharmaceutically active capsules, gels, or solutions).

Exploiting the possibility of compounding drugs in small-scale laboratories, some clinics have been producing their own hormonal implants. CEPARH has its very own farmácia de manipulação where the hormonal implants that arrive in sterile packages, which I saw implanted in the clinic, are handcrafted. Set up under the brand name Elmeco Medical and Pharmaceutical Products Ltd, this small pharmaceutical laboratory functions under the regulatory auspices of a farmácia de manipulação. It presents its mission as "serving society by producing implants with individualized doses of hormones" and explains that "Hormonal Implants offer extraordinary benefits for persons of both sexes."[4] I had the opportunity to do some fieldwork there. It is a relatively small laboratory that employs three laboratory technicians. Although hormonal implants are imagined as very high-tech treatments (a vision reinforced by advertisements in women's magazines, which set hormonal implants alongside plastic surgery and other bodily modification practices), their production is surprisingly low-tech. The manufacture of these technological objects is remarkably manual; these are quite literally handcrafted biotechnologies. The pharmacy receives rolls, several meters in length, of silicone SIL-Tec tubing. This is cut to size against a small, yellow school ruler that has been taped to the workbench. The powdered hormone, which is manually inserted into each segment of tubing, is delivered to the farmácia in opaque gray containers, kept in a row of locked cabinets, each labeled with the hormones it contains. The lab technicians explain that these are sourced from a distribuidora (retailer) in São Paulo that imports them directly from China and India, they supposed. The process of repackaging this powdered hormone into subdermal implants is labor-intensive. After cutting each tube to size, each one must be individually glued on one end and left to dry before being filled. Meanwhile, working under a vent, hormone powder is transferred from the storage containers into a mortar and pestle, where it is worked to "fluidify" the substance and make its insertion into the tubes easier. With tremendous dexterity, the tubes are dipped by bunches of five into the mortar, held and flicked with a specific gesture, an action that is repeated several times until the tube is entirely filled. An instrument

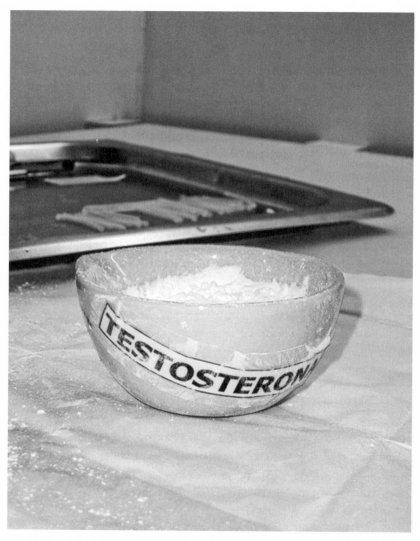

Figures 5.1 and 5.2 Handcrafting subdermal hormonal implants from powdered hormone. Photograph by Emilia Sanabria.

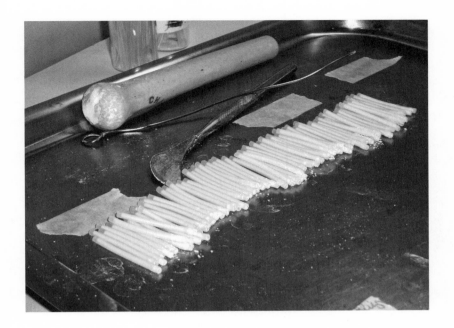

is used to pack the powder, and the tubes are weighed before the other ex-
tremity is sealed with silicone glue. Because the *substâncias* (substances, as
the technicians refer to them) have different weights, the SIL-Tec tubing
is cut to different lengths, calculated such that each implant contains fifty
milligrams of active substance, releasing four to five micrograms per day.
"Estradiol is the lightest, *não é* [obviously, isn't it]?," the senior lab techni-
cian explains, and the tubes have to be filled more tightly to obtain the correct dosage. It has a tackier consistency, she adds, and requires more work
to fill the same quantity of tubes as gestrinone or levonorgestrel. Although
both women work under a vented workbench, using gloves and a mask, they
both report having "altered cycles" and irregular bleeding patterns, which
they directly associate with their daily manipulation of hormônio.[5] Once the
tubes are filled, sealed, and quality-checked (for weight and resistance) they
are packed into plastic pouches, sterilized, and labeled. This is the form in
which they are sent up to the clinic for application by CEPARH's specially
trained nurses. Each patient receives a prescription from a doctor, and the
specifics are composed there and then from the packs sent up from the farmácia de manipulação. While presented as tailor-made, there is in actual
fact relatively little variability in the doses, although there is greater possi-

bility of dosage modulation than with other modes of hormonal administration.

Gestrinone is the most expensive, and is packed in pairs and administered by six (G6) to suppress menstruation or treat estrogen-dependent menstrual pathologies (such as endometriosis and uterine fibroids). In some patients gestrinone is associated with estradiol (e.g., E4 + G6). Elcometrine (known internationally as Nesterone) blocks estrogen and androgen peaks and is used in the treatment of polycystic ovaries or hirsutism. In combination with testosterone (1E2 + 2T) it produces fewer side effects than gestrinone, and only 30 percent of users still experience bleeding patterns after one year (Coutinho 2004).[6] Elsimar Coutinho very publicly declared at the Sixteenth Bahian Congress of Gynecology and Obstetrics that elcometrine is a particularly important hormone, given its ability to inhibit estrogen peaks. These he characterized both as dangerous to the reproductive organs and as "an embarrassment for modern women, who *exala* [give off] estrogen like a dog on heat. But unlike a dog, women do not have a tail to prevent penetration, and therefore have no natural escape. But thanks to Elcometrine, they can block their estrogen peaks."

This outrageous medicalized version of the Judeo-Christian idea that women are sexual temptresses who unleash the natural sexual urges of males proposes that self-respecting, civilized women must take (hormonal) action to curb their sexuality. This is typical of the way in which Coutinho frames the role of sex hormones in human sexuality, a vision that one of his lone public critics, Elizer Berenstein, referred to as "veterinarian" in an interview.[7] Somewhat ironically, as we have seen, sexual desire in women with low libido is simultaneously pathologized and promoted through the use of testosterone. This indicates that it is a very particular kind of sexual desire — one based on testosterone rather than estrogen — that is valued.[8] To this effect, estradiol (E2), testosterone (T), and levonorgestrel (1) are combined in a range of different combinations (6E2 + 2T; 4E2 + 3T; 6E2 + 31; 6E2 + 41, etc.) to achieve "individualized, low dose treatments, in which the bioavailability of testosterone is a crucial element in your patient's well-being," explained CEPARH's medical director, speaking at the same conference during the "Hormonal Implant Pre-Congress Course" (the most well attended course of the Sixteenth Bahian Congress of Gynecology and Obstetrics, it might be added). CEPARH's team — which count collaborators across the country — are always highly visible at national gynecological congresses, staging panels or courses during which they present the clinical indications and "advantages" of these methods. As Dr. Spinola concluded during one of SOBRAGE's (the Brazilian Society for Endocrine Gynecology) annual conferences: "hormones are good for business" because they oblige the patient to return regularly to perform many clinical exams and allow the doctor to "control her more closely." Elmeco's business is booming, and the small pharmaceutical laboratory I visited in 2006 expanded in 2011 to meet "the growing demand for its products on the national market," as the company's website explains. In August 2013 the first "National Meeting of Hormonal Implant Technologies" was hosted in Salvador by Elmeco Medical and Pharmaceutical Products Ltd. This event gathered the fifty Brazilian doctors who most prescribe hormonal implants in view of exchanging experiences and treating of themes relevant to "business" (in English on the meeting presentation website). Although I was not present at this meeting, I imagine it to be a place where—like the panels that are held to present implants to the medical profession, the media presentations of these objects, or the doctor–patient interactions where their clinical uses are discussed—particular efficacies are carved out for these evolving, labile objects. Elmeco's promotional website links directly back to http://www.elsimarcoutinho.com, where the "benefits of hormonal implants to the 'feminine public'" are presented as follows (I quote extensively, for the list is indicative of the highly idiosyncratic manner in which hormonal implants are being developed in Brazil):

- Lengthening of the vida útil [pun on dia útil, or working day, the term útil means "useful"; this thus translates as "useful" life]—social, sexual, and professional
- Decrease in risk of early death due to degenerative diseases
- Preservation of self-esteem, libido, sexuality, attraction, vaginal healthiness and lubrication, reduction of night sweats, of tiredness, improvement of cognitive functions and memory
- Maintenance of musculature, beauty, and shine of the skin and eyes, avoidance of precocious loss of hair
- Prevents and reverts osteoporosis, increases the life of the cells that build new bone, regulating the cycle of formation and absorption of osteoblasts and osteoclasts
- Diminishes the incidence of certain types of cancer, such as intestinal or endometrial cancers
- Prevention of atherosclerosis, regulation of the production of good

cholesterol (HDL), diminishing of bad cholesterol (LDL), and avoidance of heart attacks arising from accumulation of platelets
- Sex hormones are responsible for the exuding of the characteristic feminine smell, a fundamental element in sexual dynamics. Pheromones, a type of sex hormone detectable by smell, are a sub-product of testosterone and estradiol.[9]

The farmácia de manipulação where hormonal implants are handcrafted is in a small building on CEPARH's ground floor, tucked away behind a large mango tree under which the CEPARH mobile unit is parked. Two stories up, in the main building, adjacent to an air-conditioned seminar room where students from Salvador's medical faculty are taught about contraception, sexuality, and hormonal technologies, is the infirmary. This is where Renata and Solange, the specialized nurses who practice the implant insertions and removals, work. This process is relatively quick, averaging fifteen to twenty minutes, during which small talk is exchanged, often concerning the implants' effects. Patients usually come accompanied by kin—a daughter, mother, or sister. One topic that often draws discussions is the small clump of abnormally long hair-growth that regularly appears at the place of implantation, usually the *bunda* ("bum"). When spotting this, Renata never fails to exclaim: "*Veja só!* [look here!], this shows that the testosterone really works." After applying a local anesthetic, a small instrument is used to pierce into the skin a hole roughly two to three millimeters in diameter. Another instrument is used to retrieve the empty capsules, which, when examined, reveal how much of the *substância* ("substance")—as hormônio is also referred to here—is gone. Some of the tubes that are removed are not entirely empty, and traces of white residue are seen through the clear silicone tubing. This draws commentaries from patients and nurses alike, who discuss the ways in which the substâncias are absorbed, some more rapidly than others. When all capsules are completely empty before the end of the implant's normal term, Solange knowingly affirms: "You are a smoker," as smoking accelerates the rate of absorption and increases the rate at which implants need to be renewed. One patient who had come to "renew" her implants discussed the new dosage she had been prescribed with Renata, who had asked: "We are implanting something different today?" The patient explained "her" dosage had been "more tailored" because the last dose was too high and gave her *barba* (beard).

Patients often wait quite some time on the black leather sofa outside the infirmary, such that they can clearly overhear the nurses' gossip and patently see that they are not attending a patient. On one occasion, a tall, elegantly dressed woman came to have her implants renewed and was visibly fuming at having been made to wait so long and not being given an apology for the delay. She was very *sofrida* (subject to suffering/squeamish), Solange dryly remarked as her patient winced when she began extracting the empty capsules. Visibly disliking everything about the experience, the patient turned to me and exclaimed: "*Mais vale a pena que esse negocio funciona mesmo*" (But it's worth it, because this thing really works). One morning, Renata's cousin comes in and they joke about the fact that her husband has sent her because her PMT is back with a vengeance and her libido is at its lowest. Once the implants are replaced, and the small Band-Aid applied, Renata pats her on the shoulder and jokes: "*Ta chipada!*" (You're all [micro]chipped!). During São Paulo's Fashion Week 2012, a series of press articles presenting hormonal implants as *Chipes da beleza* (beauty chips) were released, including coverage in Brazil's leading broadsheet A Folha de Sao Paulo. This article explains that hormonal implants are appreciated by models as a convenient form of contraception that also suppresses menstruation, regulates premenstrual tension, pain, and swelling, diminishes cellulite, and avoids weight gain (Bilenky 2012). The only problem with the "hormonal chip," states Brazilian model Natália Zambiasi, is that "it makes you *tarada* [a sex maniac]." Footballer Ronaldo's ex-girlfriend, model Raica Oliveira, explains she used implants for eight years and is eager to renew them because without them "I need to work out more, my bum is sagging; when I use the implant it is all firm and hard." Ford Model Talytha Pugliesi states: "First you de-swell, then you *dá uma secada* [dry out or lose weight], lose cellulite, gain muscle, your body becomes firmer and your skin texture improves. Plus you free yourself of menstruation!" Covergirl Thaís Rumpel, aged seventeen, was sent to Montgomery's private practice by her agency (Ford Models Brasil). "Before using the 'chip' my hormones were all disorganized and I would gain weight and fluctuate a lot," she explains. The agency is reported to have made the advance payment of US$1,000 that the model will reimburse. ELO modeling agency director Renata Rodrigues confirms the existence of partnerships between modeling agencies and Montgomery's or Coutinho's clinics. More than 1 million doses were applied in Brazil in 2011 according to Coutinho (Bilenky 2012).

On another morning observing implant insertions, a patient entered the small infirmary and was greeted by Renata, who exclaimed: "*Você sumiu que-*

rida!" (You had disappeared, darling!), asking her what had kept her away for so long. "I had to have everything removed: my uterus, my ovaries, the whole lot. Now that *ta tudo tranquilo* [all's in order] I'm back," the patient explained. This example, while extreme, points to the ways in which, in Salvador, these treatments do not necessarily follow strict treatment categorizations (as contraceptive treatments, treatments for hormone replacement therapy, and so on) but often blur indications. The implants this patient was having were—in dosage—analogous to a prescription given to a woman to "treat" her menstrual disorders. Because of her relatively young age, Renata did not refer to it as "replacement," but as the patient left she said to her: "*Você va ver, va dar uma boa equilibrada*" (You'll see, it will give you a good balancing out). Maria do Carmen is a stunning fifty-seven-year-old woman, elegantly dressed, her hair straightened and her long red nails immaculate. She has been using hormonal implants ever since she discovered her husband's affair, she tells us one morning, as Solange applies the anesthetic and begins the implant renewal procedure. They are both widowed and have been married over twenty years. They have a total of twelve children, from previous marriages, most of whom are settled. Her husband, who travels to São Paulo regularly for work, was given testosterone to treat his impotence, she explains. He started to want sex all the time. "*Eu não tinha condição, nem vontade*" (I didn't have the conditions, nor the desire), she remarks. When he stopped insisting, she thought the treatment was wearing off, but then discovered that he was sleeping with their domestic employee, who is younger than her eldest daughter, she added. "I cried for days," she explains. "We made up. He changed, he is attentive again. I have been using implants and I have to say, they really help." Solange nods approvingly. "*Tem que se cuidar mesmo*" (You really do have to care for yourself), she agrees.

The stories that are exchanged during this process struck me in the ways they attribute specific efficacies to sex hormones. Observing the empty capsules removed from their bodies as evidence of the experience that their effects had worn out, these women made very direct connections between the materials that their bodies expunged from the capsules and the discursively reinforced sets of experiences attributed to different hormones. These hormonal efficacies are, in turn, heavily reinforced through the mediatized discourses of doctors in the women's press and on social media. Selfies of patients with their implant-prescribing doctors abound on Instagram followed by a series of hashtags such as #doctor's name, #hormone name, *#amo* (#love), *#mudominhavida* (#changedmylife), *#parabenspeloseutrabalho*

(#congratulationsforyourwork), *#indicacaoatodasmulheres* (#recommended-toallwomen). The Brazilian *Marie Claire* edition ran a feature on the "Magic of Hormones," which outlines the role of different hormones in "our happiness."[10] "In the first two weeks of the menstrual cycle, when the brain is swimming in estrogens, eroticism and femininity are at their peak, and general disposition is good. Then, under the influence of progesterone, women become more sensitive, introspective and sometimes feel irritation," an endocrinologist from São Paulo explains. The feature presents estrogen as the "Emperor of Sex," and as lowering stress, favoring skin tones, and stimulating "active sexual desire" and "sensuality," as well as good humor and mental clarity and regulating metabolism. A cover story in the Brazilian women's magazine *Boa Forma*'s (Good Shape) column *Famosas em Boa Forma* (Stars in Good Shape) reported that telenovela actress Carla Regina had recently lost five kilograms.[11] In the column she explains that her boyfriend, gynecologist Malcolm Montgomery, provided invaluable help by prescribing tailored hormonal implants. Montgomery, as we saw in the introduction, is more famous for his regular appearances in people magazines than for his scientific publications (which are few and far between). In the Regina "news" coverage, he explains that he switched "Carla's" implants because the previous testosterone combination "injected protein into her muscles augmenting their volume. The new combination removes excess swelling and thins her silhouette." Montgomery is quoted as adding that "hormonal implants should not be adopted just for weight loss as their prime medical function is to control hormonal fluctuations and reduce menstrual episodes," but "the specialist"—as he is presented—notes that they also have "this interesting aesthetic effect." An article published in the wake of the widespread coverage the *Chipes da beleza* received during São Paulo's Fashion Week 2012 noted that Brazil's Federal Council of Medicine does not recommend the use of implants for "esthetic ends."[12] The Brazilian Society for Endocrinology and Metabolism does not support the uses developed nationally for these hormonal compounds. However, as we have seen, a parallel society called the Brazilian Society for Endocrine Gynecology (presided by members of CEPARH and associated clinics in São Paulo) actively promotes the development of implant prescriptions through specific congresses, events, and panels in mainstream medical congresses. Although it is legal to import elcometrin and gestrinone, their sale in pharmacies is prohibited, as is—formally—their commercialization in implants. The private clinics that are delivering these methods and actively promoting them through the media are operating through a legal loophole, given that their legal register with Brazil's pharmacovigilance institution ANVISA expired nearly a decade ago. ANVISA recently issued a statement to say that several establishments that had been commercializing the drugs illegally had been fined, and had initiated a legal appeal—a rather classic situation in Brazil. In the wait for a formal legal resolution, doctors continue to combine—somewhat experimentally—different doses, adding or removing estrogen or testosterone rods to produce the desired effects.

Problem of Evanescent Objecthood

The blurred indications and local uses of these labile drugs trouble the relationship between the stabilized drug form and the uses they are approved for in other regions of the world. In Brazil, as we have seen, contraceptive injections or Mirena are commonly used to stop menstruating, oral contraceptive pills such as Yasmin and its national copies are used to "lose" weight, and hormonal implants are used to "replace" or "balance" hormones, thereby boosting sexual desire and *disposição* or reducing emotional fluctuations, irrespective of whether they are primarily adopted as contraceptives. Unlike in Western Europe or North America, where regulation seeks to limit such blurring of therapeutic indications, in Brazil there is greater institutional and legal flexibility around these uses. This flexibility has meant that drugs are circulated, fractioned, combined, and repackaged with far greater ease there. There would be a great deal more to say about this, in contrast, for example, to how population-level risks of hormonal contraceptives are or not constructed in different national contexts, to the role of national and private insurance in defining levels of reimbursement or coverage, and in the way private and public health are intermeshed in Brazil.[13] For the present purposes, however, I wish to point to the way that regulatory practices contribute to further packaging (and to some extent black-boxing) the social labor that goes into producing these things into stabilized objects. This is to say that to ask about the indications or social profile of a drug overlooks the painstaking labor involved in getting from an active principle to a regime of proof concerning a specific therapeutic efficacy to a marketable product and branded drug entity. The anthropological literature on the pharmaceutical copy (Greene 2011; Hayden 2007, 2013; Sunder Rajan, forthcoming) points to the stakes involved—for the pharmaceutical industry and for nation-states defending national industries—in maintaining the black-box closed, in keeping the object tightly bounded together, to protect research and development (and, one might add, marketing) investments that have produced the thing as an object. This literature examines how, with the proliferations taking place on the side of the copy, the tight relationship that is crafted between an active principle and branded, packaged drug entities was destabilized. Greenslit's (2005) work on Sarafem (Prozac "re-packaged" for premenstrual dysphoric disorder) reveals the way that, in the United States, physicians are informed that Sarafem and Prozac are the same drug in different packaging, whereas patient information emphasizes that these are different drugs with the same ingredient (481). What the paper reveals is that drug categories are increasingly determined not by their chemical makeup, but by their brand, that is, by the marketing strategies that produce them as (packaged) products. This provides an interesting counterexample to the ways in which hormones are repackaged in Salvador, for in the range of uses that are made of these extremely labile objects, it is clear that neither drug entities nor disease identities are ever clear-cut. Thus, unlike the U.S. contexts, where considerable efforts are deployed to associate trademarked products with a given "clinical entity," in the context that I know, this stabilization of the relation between drug and clinical entity is not subject to the same degree of explicit negotiation. Observing the way contraceptive sex hormones are repackaged in Brazil, in a context where regulatory practices are less stringent, sheds light, through its absence, on the work of holding things stable as bounded objects. My point is that we often have, in anthropological studies of pharmaceuticals, taken the object for granted. Taking the object for granted in this context refers to the way assumptions are made about the relation between the form of the object and its function. Over the course of presenting my findings, I have often been asked whether hormonal implants or injections are contraceptives or lifestyle drugs, whether extended-regime oral contraceptive pills aim to treat menstrual problems or reduce the number of periods women experience. These questions reproduce a logic in which a drug is approved for a given indication and overlook the highly dynamic way in which primary and secondary effects are continuously reworked by users, doctors, and marketers. They assume the existence of regulatory practices that distinguish between these functions and effects and overlook the fact that in many regions of the world institutions that perform this regulatory work are direly absent.[14]

During my fieldwork, the body of literature known as "pharmaceutical anthropology" proved incredibly helpful, both theoretically and methodologically, because it allowed me to move beyond a hospital-focused ethnography to a community-focused one, and to follow the social life of these objects as they moved between domains that are often kept apart in anthropological analyses. In *Social Lives of Medicines* (Whyte, van der Geest, and Hardon 2002) the authors propose that the importance of considering medicines as material culture is twofold. It is, they argue, "the 'thinginess' of medicines and their tendency to become commodities" that suit them to an analysis as objects of material culture. The materiality of medicines, it is argued, is of great importance to anthropology, for it is as objects that medicines are exchanged, and that anthropologists can map their biographies and careers through a range of social contexts. It is also as material objects that they "objectify meanings" (5). Whyte et al. (2002) are concerned with elucidating the ways in which drugs are made efficacious. Efficacy, they show, is "multifaceted" (33). While biomedicine tends to define efficacy as a property of the drug (its active principles), anthropological work on pharmaceuticals reveals that the way people perceive drugs—even pharmaceutically inert drugs such as placebos—plays a role in their potential to be efficacious. This is something that Moerman (2002, 56) called "the meaning response," to refer to the ways in which the symbolic exerts its influence over the biological. In addition to the meaning response, Whyte et al. (2002) outline "social efficacy," which includes the relational context within which medicines are made meaningful and efficacy is coconstructed by patients, health providers, and kin. The "total effect," they argue, is the product of the interplay between the biochemical properties of drugs and the social, cultural, and symbolic effects that they bare in excess to these. While these are all important considerations, they do little to explain exactly *how* objects "concretize" illness and cure. Thus, the authors argue: "The problem of efficacy relates to perceptions of the powers of medicinal substances. This brings us to the symbolic nature of medicines and the question of not what, but how, medicines mean. . . . When medicinal substances with such meaningful associations are applied to ailing bodies, they concretize the problem, and thus make it accessible to therapeutic action of a fitting symbolic nature. Suggesting connections and making disorder and its correction tangible is the symbolic and very practical work of medicines, even those synthesized in factories and prescribed by doctors" (Whyte et al. 2002, 15).

Despite the promise of this approach as a whole, the analysis of the therapeutic efficacy of drugs at times reproduces distinctions between the material and the social, or the symbolic. In reverting to the notion of the symbolic power of medicines, for example, the authors situate their analysis within a representational mode in which meaning is tagged onto things, or in which things and meanings are taken to be of different orders.[15] Although approaching pharmaceuticals as material objects is extremely useful, such analyses overlook two aspects of drugs' materiality that I would like to focus on here. The first concerns the various ways in which pharmacologically active principles are turned into pharmaceutical commodities of the kinds that are exchanged. The second examines the relationship between the form given to these objects and their consumption. My suggestion is that the analytic possibilities afforded by the *social life of medicines* approach are not always fully realized because the unity or givenness of these objects is at times taken for granted. Making pharmaceutical substances into drugs (objects that can circulate) is an elaborate process, the analysis of which can illuminate something of the politics of object making in contemporary Euro-American practices. In calling attention to the ways in which these objects are crafted and transformed, I want to comment more generally on what Appadurai (2006) called "the fragility of objecthood." The point of interest is that these objects don't just come undone at the seams when we look at their *making*. What is particular about pharmaceuticals is that their efficacy is entirely dependent on their dissolution and absorption. They are objects that are destined to disappear and to dissolve, and their production as objects aims to maximize this ultimate dispersal. Yet form is centrally important, if highly transient in this context. This material transposition from self-contained object of public attention to dissolved therapeutic in the body alerts us to the political significance of the boundaries that delimit the states of being of a medical commodity. This is something I have referred to as the evanescent aspects of pharmaceuticals (Sanabria 2010).

The practices of the manipulation pharmacy make explicit a process that is often overlooked in analyses of pharmaceuticals as objects: namely their production and stabilization into objects out of their various constitutive materials. This is largely because, as anthropologists, we usually encounter them ready-bounded and packaged. My work on the recontextualizations and repackagings of sex hormones has led me to question the unity and boundedness of these things in their form as pharmaceuticals, because of the extraordinary profusion of forms in which these objects come and guises under which I encountered them in the course of fieldwork. The production of this diversity was, as we saw at the outset of the chapter, fueled by attempts to make these objects more consumable by more users. This consumable aspect of drugs, to which I now turn, is one that has received less attention in anthropology, despite holding the potential for new ways of conceiving of pharmaceutical efficacies. Anthropological studies of consumption tend, by in large, not to study consumption in the sense of "using up of a material," "making away with," "take up and exhaust as material," and "reduce to invisible products" (all *Oxford English Dictionary* definitions), but to focus instead on why certain objects are consumed (as in sought and acquired) rather than others. Patterns of consumption—as in acquisition—and the social structures these reflect occupy the vast majority of these studies. Yet the materiality of consumption in its primary meaning would merit greater attention. As it stands, the models available to think through the circulation, acquisition, and consumption of objects seem to take us only up to the moment at which these things are consumed (as in digested and absorbed). There is less of a focus on the degradation, rotting, dissolution, desegregation, or other metamorphoses of the objects that capture our attention. This is a point that Ingold (2007) makes when he argues that material culture focuses on the "materiality of *objects*" without giving sufficient consideration to *materials* and their properties: "For such studies take as their starting point a world of objects that has, as it were, already crystallised out of the fluxes of materials and their transformations. At this point materials appear to vanish, swallowed up by the very objects to which they gave birth. That is why we commonly describe materials as 'raw' but never 'cooked'—for by the time they have congealed into objects they have already disappeared. Henceforth it is the objects themselves that capture our attention, no longer the materials of which they are made" (9).

This carves out a particular place for pharmaceuticals in the analysis of material things, and of material culture in the analysis of pharmaceuticals—something that has been overlooked by both bodies of literature. While material culture initially seemed to provide elements to theorize pharmaceuticals as "things," the consumable and changeable aspect of these things is often undertheorized. Ingold levels an important critique to actor–network theories (ANT), one which is of particular interest to medical anthropologists who seek to account for the ways in which bodies encounter healing techniques of varying kinds. While I tend to be less severe in my assessments of ANT than Ingold is, I find his suggestion that such theories are limited by the fact that they often focus predominantly on inert, inorganic, or man-made nonhumans both true and useful. The first to level this critique at Latour was Haraway (1992, n14), when she noted the importance of thinking with animals and other nonmachine nonhumans when theorizing nonhumans. Ingold has more recently called for a turn to materials in an attempt to move past the preboundedness that the concepts of "materiality" and "object" have acquired in material culture studies (Ingold 2007). Like Haraway, Ingold (2012, 436) is concerned that Latour's nonhumans are "resolutely inanimate." Material culture studies, he argues, operate with a conception of the material world that "focuses on the artefactual domain at the expense of living organisms" (428). This omission of organic life-forms and the material processes responsible for growth, decay, rotting, or non-human-induced transformations of the material world is a key blind spot that Ingold reveals in the way anthropologists and social theorists more generally engage with the material world. For this reason, he strategically mobilizes—with Heidegger—the term *thing* contra *object*: "The object stands before us as a *fait accompli*, presenting its congealed, outer surfaces to our inspection. . . . The thing, by contrast . . . has the character not of an externally bounded entity, set over and against the world, but of a knot whose constituent threads, far from being contained within it, trail beyond, only to become caught with other threads in other knots. Or in a word, things leak, forever discharging through the surfaces that form temporarily around them" (Ingold 2010, 4).

Ingold's project (2007, 2012) is to rethink phenomenology through material culture. Bodies breathe, grow, decay, and their existence depends on their ability to incorporate their environments through the acquisition of skills or nourishment that travel across their "ever-emergent surfaces."

> The living body, likewise, is sustained thanks only to the continual taking in of materials from its surroundings and, in turn, the discharge into them, in the processes of respiration and metabolism. Things can exist and persist only because they *leak*: that is, because of the inter-change of materials across the ever-emergent surfaces by which they differentiate themselves from the surrounding medium. The bodies of organisms and other things leak continually; indeed, their lives depend on it. Precisely this shift of perspective from stopped-up objects to leaky things distinguishes the ecology of materials from mainstream studies of material culture. (Ingold 2012, 438)

If such objects are conceptualized as lively, leaky *things* rather than stopped-up entities, positing their agency is unnecessary. Their embroilment in flows of transformation does not require a theory of how they come to "act." This point is important when considering the efficacy of drugs, for drugs are things that work *in* bodies specifically through their leakiness. What drugs do, their agency as material objects (which medical anthropologists have studied as "effects"), is made possible only in living bodies. Their bioavailabilities are not the sole property of the things themselves but of these things in relation to living, metabolizing bodies. In this sense pharmaceutical drugs are very specific kinds of *things*. My aim in mobilizing Ingold here is to suggest ways of thinking about how to move beyond analyses that posit a dual form of efficacy for drugs: a biomedical one (that is at times unquestioned) and a symbolic one (whose capacity to produce tangible biological effects is stated but seldom explained). My suggestion is not that we dismiss symbolic efficacies but rather that we explore in more detail how the symbolic and the material become enmeshed, reinforcing and strengthening one another in such ways as to make it ever more difficult to say where one begins and the other ends. In what follows I argue that marketing and the discourses relayed through the media, doctor–patient interactions, and informal exchanges of information on drug regimens among kin and peers serve to weave together these varied efficacies in intricate and powerful ways.

On several occasions, Schering's regional representative, Anderson, took me out "to visit his gynecologists." The private practices in Anderson's clientele are luxurious, their interior design mixing white marble floors, spotless glass doors, and colorful popular art. Schering's products are considered *muito chique* (very chic), as one gynecologist put it. Anderson engages the conversation with the doctor as an equal, taking his time, making a few jokes. He knows his products matter here. He is here to "defend" Yasmin, one of Brazil's leading brands containing the fourth-generation hormone drospirenone, meticulously marketed by Schering, as we have seen, as the *bem-estar* (well-being) pill, for it is presented as reducing swelling and weight gain, given the diuretic effects of drospirenone. Several national laboratories have launched "copies" (both generic and nongeneric *similares*, as they are referred to locally), and Schering is concerned about patent infringement and the loss of market this entails.[16] "*Doctora*, I want you to help me make Yasmin the number one option for your patients. It's the best product on the market: it's about your patient's well-being. She won't experience that swelling that makes her swap. And Yasmin is the real thing, the guarantee of quality, not just a copy."

In 2012 the Brazilian laboratory EMS Sigma Farma launched several pills containing drospirenone. EMS's marketing strategy is explicitly founded on promising *more*: "More beauty, more lightness and more freedom for *more* women," as its drospirenone copy retails at roughly half the price of Yasmin. The way hormonal contraceptives are experienced depends on a subtle balance of tangible and intangible elements, which include—beyond the chemical composition of a drug—attention to aspects of the brand, such as design, logo, name, image, and, increasingly, the concept. In a context where direct-to-consumer advertising cannot publicize specific brand names, modes of administration have become key elements of the branded concept, such as "Discover implantable contraception" (Implanon); "Oh! Once-a-month birth control" (Nuvaring); "Fewer Periods. More Possibilities." (Seasonale); and "Keep life simple. Birth control for busy moms" (Mirena). These are, in turn, associated with specific color ranges, fonts, symbols, and keywords. The concepts that a brand carries, such as that of well-being and weight loss, widely associated with Yasmin through extensive marketing campaigns in Brazil, seep into the hormonal substance itself: drospirenone, in this case. Thus, aspects of a brand may percolate unevenly to the copies of the chemical compounds as these are remade under new guises, packagings, or as they are copied by generic manufacturers.

Modifications in the mode of administration induce changes in the perception and experience procured by the object that may be so significant that they eclipse the common hormonal action between two drugs. Where hormonal implant and Mirena are concerned, many of the users I interviewed explicitly rejected any association between these and the pill.[17] To some extent, biomedical technologies such as Mirena or hormonal implants cease to appear as drugs, despite their pharmacological action. Marketing for Mirena somewhat downplays its hormonal action, with discursive attention being held in the fact that it is an intrauterine device. It is therefore more understandable that this method be less associated with its hormonal action. However, hormonal implants are widely appreciated for their menstrual-suppressive action, and much of the promotion of this method centers on controlling the hormonal fluxes associated with premenstrual tension. This is because the marketing of contraceptives invites users to think of methods less in terms of their constitutive pharmacological properties, and more in terms of their mode of administration. For example, Nara runs a small business and has been using Mirena for two years. She is twenty-nine and has a daughter of four who lives with her and her parents in a modern high-rise building. As a busy working mother, Nara appreciates not having to think about contraception daily. Her contraceptive history is marked by what she calls an "erratic" use of the pill. Her pregnancy was unplanned and, following an abortion three years later, she used a copper IUD. This gave her painful and heavy periods, and she became aware of having what she describes as "tremendous" premenstrual tension. Her gynecologist suggested Mirena, which is often prescribed in such cases, and her partner helped her meet the cost, which amounted to over US$250. She explains that she never "got on" well with hormones, despite the fact that Mirena has a hormonal delivery system and that she enjoys the fact that Mirena suppresses her period. When I press her on this she laughs, stating that "it's totally different." This can be explained by the fact that Nara adopted Mirena specifically as an alternative to the pill: "I went for it as an *anticoncepcional* [contraceptive], to be free to travel and everything without having to depend on a pill. And I got on well with it. And on top of everything, I stopped menstruating, then I was really loving it."

Likewise, Simone has been using hormonal implants for six years because she dislikes the pill. She is a professional photographer and runs a large events business. Simone, who is vegan, a yogi, and makes use of a range of holistic therapies such as Reiki, explains that she never uses medications and prefers to heal herself through meditation or by attending to the meaning that a particular physical ailment is conveying. She speaks of loving her implants in terms of a "confession," explaining that they give her tremendous "disposition" for life but that she worries "about what it might be doing to my organism. I love it, but I'm scared of using another one." She recognizes the hormonal composition of her implants and its risks, and appreciates the effects of the testosterone that heightens her *tesão* (sexual desire) and gives her extra physical strength, but she clearly differentiates the implant from the pill—which she notes is more highly dosed—or the morning-after pill that she describes as a "hormonal bomb." Beyond its practicality as a contraceptive, this method seems to Simone to be less of a biomedical intervention, in that she does not have to take a pill every day, a fact that sits more easily with her holistic vision of health (despite the fact that she no longer experiences menstrual periods). However, it enables her to sustain her demanding lifestyle and meet her professional and social obligations unencumbered by what she calls "emotional disruptions" or "menstrual *fraqueza* [weakness]."

Beyond facilitating use and overcoming forgetfulness, nonoral sex hormone repackaging strategies bear directly on the bioavailability of an active principle in the body. When a drug is swallowed and absorbed by the digestive system, it is metabolized by the liver. As we have seen, this reduces the bioavailability of the drug, requiring the administration of a higher dose. Alternative routes of administration avoid so-called first-pass[18] effects through their delivery directly into the circulatory system. Differences of these kinds have important ramifications on the way an otherwise similar chemical compound acts in the body. Users' subjective experiences of a drug's efficacy are thus mediated by a range of factors that include its active principle, its mode of administration—which in turn determines the drug's pharmacokinetics—and the social context within which it is prescribed and consumed. The cases discussed here reveal new fault lines through which the *pharmakon* exerts it influence, collapsing the distinctions between biological and sociological factors. The attention the industry places on pharmacodynamics suggests ways in which effects are already both biological and social, symbolic and experienced in the flesh. In repeatedly alluding to differences in the *effects* of nonoral methods, these women are speaking at one and the same time of differences in the rates and magnitudes of pharmacologic responses, in the quotidian practices of use, and in the medical encounters where these methods are prescribed—as well as ensuing differences in the subjective identities locally conferred by "having an implant" or "using Mirena." These cases reveal how different the same thing, repackaged, can look and *feel*. They point to what can be gained by considering pharmaceutical efficacy as the cumulative effect of the reputation, appearance, or subjective attachments to specific drugs, to their brands, pharmaceutical formulations and modes of administration, as well as to the social contexts within which drugs are used.

Conclusion

Considering pharmaceuticals as objects was a conceptually and methodologically important move. However, it produced a blind spot, which concerns the givenness of the object status of pharmaceuticals. I have sought to bring attention to the powerfully reinforcing relationships between active principles, form or mode of administration, discursive elements that accompany the delivery of a specific drug, and the ensuing embodied effects that are (or are not) associated by users with the substance they have consumed. The pharmaceutical industry's repackaging strategies aim to enhance drug delivery by offering novel pathways of administration. Nonoral modes of hormonal administration, for example, aim both to circumvent first-pass metabolism by the liver (a biochemical and clinical concern) and to increase patient reliability, or minimize user "failure" or "forgetfulness." Here, biochemical and biopolitical concerns intermingle. The changes made to the form of pharmaceutical objects—inasmuch as we can hold the object stable analytically—are intrinsically linked to the ways in which these objects perform their central function, which is to successfully dissolve and disappear. Heeding greater attention to the changeable, perishable, or transformable aspects of things highlights the sociocultural practices that reenact them as bounded or stable entities. This approach sets out a specific role for the anthropological inquiry into the realm of pharmaceutical artefacts as it provides a frame to think about the different objects enacted, not as different meanings or interpretations of the ostensibly underlying real object, but as different enactments (material and social) of these objects.

Feminist philosopher of science Karen Barad (2007) proposes some useful conceptual vocabulary with which to overcome the view that we can neatly separate matter from the interpretation of matter. Objects, Barad (2007, 127) tells us, drawing on her double expertise as a physicist and critical social theorist, do not have an ontology independent of the conditions of determinability specified by the apparatus through which they are known. "Since individually determinate entities do not exist, measurements do not entail an interaction between separate entities; rather, determinate entities emerge from their intra-action. I introduce the term 'intra-action' in recognition of their ontological inseparability, in contrast to the usual 'interaction,' which relies on a metaphysics of individualism (in particular, the prior existence of separately determinate entities). A phenomenon is a specific intra-action of an 'object' and the 'measuring agencies'; the object and the measuring agencies emerge from, rather than precede, the intra-action that produces them" (128).

This enables her to postulate that phenomena are real physical entities without having to postulate that they exist outside the dynamic topological entanglements and relationalities that articulate them (141). "A lively new ontology emerges: the world's radical aliveness comes to light in an entirely nontraditional way that reworks the nature of both relationality and aliveness (vitality, dynamisms, agency)," she concludes (33). This ontology is rather different from one that purports to bring matter back in while continuing to radically differentiate between the discursive, cultural, or symbolic on one hand and the material on the other (see Mol 2013, 380). I draw on Barad here to argue that there can be no knowledge of hormonal effects outside the practices that make these known and the bodies that experience them and report on these experiences. The point is a deceptively simple one, for accounting for hormonal effects is particularly tricky business. While their effects may be widely shared—albeit with significant cross-cultural variation, as Lock (1993) has forcefully demonstrated—there is little medical consensus concerning their effects. The role of hormones in the premenstrual syndrome or in bringing about weight gain or subjective/cognitive effects of the kinds I have reported here is widely disputed in the medical literature and by many medical professionals, despite the fact that countless users report such effects. Likewise, their clinically attested efficacy as aphrodisiacs is contested, a point that Hoberman (2005) makes in his cultural history of testosterone, although there is a booming global market for such indications. It is therefore useful to consider such effects through the lens of intra-action. This concept helps us move past the idea that there is a real underlying reality that discourses (or the evidentiary practices of clinical trials demonstrating therapeutic efficacies) more or less aptly "reveal." In this chapter I have suggested that we attend to the production—both conceptual and technical—of hormones and examine the practices that give them their contour as recognizable, nameable, agentic entities (Barad 2007). This is to say that matter actively participates in the production of phenomena (in the sense given by Barad); it "kicks back." Thinking hormonal effects through the lens of intra-action makes it nonsensical to ask whether the efficacy is biological or the product of branding, cultural evaluations of efficacy, the meaningfulness of therapeutic encounters, or "placebo effects." The effects of hormones—and of other drugs—cannot be reduced to their sole pharmacological action. Their gendered, contraceptive, or cognitive effects are entirely dependent on complex global infrastructures, clinical practices, knowledge production technologies, the logics of branding, the design of administration regimes, *and* the active principles that are absorbed into myriad bodies in highly diverse social settings.

CONCLUSION

LIMITS THAT DO NOT FORECLOSE

Bodies in Analogic Traffic

This book has sought to trace the mutually constitutive coming-into-beings of bodies and hormones in Bahia. It has done so through a focus on the embodied experience of menstruation and its hormonal suppression and an analysis of how blood emerges as a locus upon and through which varying types of effects (chemical, affective, relational, infectious, metaphysical) infold themselves into bodies. My analysis of menstruation in Bahia introduces a central theme that runs through the book, namely the question of how boundaries—and bodily boundaries, in particular—are sustained, negotiated, or made porous. Drawing on interview data on menstruation and hormone use, I examined the different ways Bahian women experience and deal with menstrual cycle changes. Rather than presenting hormonal menstrual suppression as an entirely novel phenomenon, I set this practice alongside strategies of menstrual management that have long been available to women. In Bahia, menstruation is widely discussed in terms of its naturalness or artificiality. I therefore set out to examine the idea that women should be able to choose if and when to menstruate in light of the reasons they give for their choice. The practice appeals to an ideal of modernity, emblematized by a move out of nature made possible through technological intervention. I pursued my analysis of the role of sex hormones in practices of bodily transformation in Brazil by showing how sex hormones are mobilized as modes of regulatory control on the one hand and to discipline individuals on the other. With the circulation of pharmaceutical sex hormones, a key aspect of sex—that defined by hormonal action—is now partially exogenous to the body. This led me to consider the relative plasticity of sexual identities and the role of sex hormones in facilitating transformations of these identities. The production of sex hormones into drugs stabilized these objects, giving substance to a set of medical ideas. I thus suggested that we attend to the materiality of drugs beyond their pharmaceutical composition when considering their effects. The focus has been on the uses of chemicals to modulate bodies and affective states. I am well aware that this has produced a vision of plasticity and malleability perhaps at times marked by an overly promissory tone. Yet, as Michelle Murphy (2011, 34) acutely reminds us: "As already chemically saturated beings, already changed and not just potentially or intentionally malleable, the ontological politics of reproduction turns on this problem of alterability. The politics of alterability is not just a question of what change to choose. It is also a politics of the differential availability of alteration to stratified subjects, alterations that can be unwanted and not just wanted, that can be life-taking and not just life-fostering."

Part of the problem stems from the fact that I have truncated this analysis to purposeful engagements with chemicals, only partially heeding to my own call to follow the things through their diverse leakages. While I have attempted to demonstrate the pervasiveness of the idea that steroid hormones affect perception, disposition, gendered sense of self, sexual desire, reproductive capacities, vitality, and energy levels, I have paid less attention to the horizon of toxic environmental effects that I would likely have found if I had made my questions about them more pressing. As chemicals are absorbed into human metabolisms and leaked back out into postindustrial water cycles (Fortun 2012), to be traced across the organisms that make up the ecological webs of relatedness in which humans are embedded, they trouble and reconfigure topological spaces. In this book my primary concern has been with troubling bodily topologies—between inside and out—and with the corrosive effects that chemicals have for our theoretical constructs.[1] In mapping their dissolution or leakage, the bodies that they encounter and the spaces they occupy begin to appear less clearly demarcated, more infolded. If we follow the materials, we need to step outside the theoretical constructs through which they leak. This points to a methodological horizon beyond the multisited (Marcus 1995), one that explicitly connects the synthetic chemicals at the heart of the pharmaceutical assemblage and those that are only beginning to enter the scope of global health's concern with environmental health. New work is emerging that attempts to think these witting and unwitting efficacies together, from the carcinogenic side effects of the massive global health rollout of antiretrovirals to toxic capital (Livingstone 2012), or that explicitly ties the defense of national welfare infrastructure to reduced environmental regulation and tax breaks for petroleum-dependent industries that saturate environments with toxic waste (Murphy 2011). Following materials (versus following objects) implies more than multisituatedness. It problematizes the notion of locality and connectedness (Yates-Doerr 2014, 2015). It also challenges us to think about what is (made) invisible, unknowable, or unmeasurable. Murphy (2008, 701) has shown that tracking the entangled and enfolded political economy of molecular relations requires an attention to the way the stratified distribution of toxicity produces new forms of precariousness. "Not only are we experiencing new forms of chemical embodiment that molecularly tie us to local and transnational economies, but so too processed food, hormonally altered meat, and pesticide-dependent crops become the material sustenance of humanity's molecular recomposition. We are further altered by the pharmaceuticals imbibed at record-profit rates, which are then excreted half metabolized back into the sewer to flow back to local bodies of water, and then again redispersed to the populace en masse through the tap. In the twenty-first century, humans are chemically transformed beings" (696).

Plastic Bodies traces how, in the Bahian biomedical landscape I have described, women come to understand themselves as chemically transformed and transformable beings. Hormone use, as we have seen, reveals the tentativeness of the boundary between "naturally" occurring hormonal fluxes and those modulated by pharmacological adjunction. Menstrual suppression, as a chemical means of "choosing nature," is a peculiar kind of purification. Regular menstruation is a typical hybrid: It is, as we have seen, the product of sociomaterial practices. The twenty-eight-day "normal" menstrual cycle experienced by pill users is itself a sociotechnical invention, produced by the stabilization of the 21/7 pill regimen. Likewise, the occurrence of regular menstrual episodes is affected by food availability, the copresence of other women, child-spacing strategies, or hormone use. As one woman astutely noted in an interview: "Everything *meixe* [mixes/interferes] with menstruation, stress, yoga, work and all the little things of the everyday." Hormonal menstrual suppression explicitly recognizes the hybrid quality of menstruation and seeks to purify this through the rationale of a technical return to nature. The appeal to the distinction between nature and intervention—or artifice—carries, in Brazil, particular values concerning modernity and the nation. Rose and Novas (2006, 442) argued that contemporary developments in "biological citizenship" transform understandings of biology as destiny, making the biological mutable, improvable, and "eminently manipulable." This is a key aspect of the new regime of biopolitics, according to Rose (2007, 40), opening up infinite possibilities for intervention: "Our somatic, corporeal, neurochemical individuality now becomes a field of choice, prudence, and responsibility. It is opened up to experimentation and contestation. Life is not imagined as an unalterable fixed endowment. *Biology is no longer destiny*. . . . It is no longer possible to sustain the line of differentiation between interventions targeting susceptibility to illness or frailty on the one hand, and interventions aimed at the enhancement of capacities on the other" (emphasis added).

Rose reveals how Euro-Americans discover this in the twenty-first-century mode of biopolitics, but as I have shown throughout the book, this is not entirely new in the Brazilian context. The material presented here clearly suggests that although the body occupies a prominent place in Brazilian social life, it is not imagined as a piece of nature, or as fixed and immutable. On the contrary. What my material reveals is that this shift in the way people come to (re)assess the relationship between nature and culture is not dependent on the development of the novel techniques that these authors describe. The natural is already intervened in; nature is already understood as plastic, as it were.

We may trace this historically to the social hygienism of the interwar period, which helped to supplant traditional religious and patriarchal codes of conduct with an infinitely variable hygienic one; or relate it, as I have intimated, to the specific value invested in all things improved and enhanced. This might account for the fact that in Bahian women's narratives, biomedical interventions rarely allude to a return to an original state of nature, as tends to be the case in accounts we are given of bodily modification in Western European or North American contexts. Feminist philosopher Heyes (2007, 17) analyzes a range of normalizing techniques of self-transformation, showing how "almost every body is now 'failed' in some respect." In the North American context she describes, the discourse of somatic individuality hinges on a distinction between inner and outer self, in which the former is conceptually prior to the latter: "Through working on the body, the inner truth of the self can be displayed, and painful moments of false recognition can be avoided: the transsexual is a man trapped in a woman's body . . . the dieter is a moderate, well-disciplined, and hardworking person, whose moral character deserves to be read from her slender form: the recipient of cosmetic surgery is 'beautiful inside'" (23).

In Bahia I seldom heard this language of self-authenticity, of returning to something original, located inside, and the body is rarely narrated as the depository of an original identity. Instead, practices of self-transformation are productive; they reveal the body to be a field of potentiality. The language is that of activating potential, not returning to something pure, something before. This is perhaps best captured in the common Brazilian idiom of being *produzida* (produced, usually in the feminine). Produzida refers to the elaborate panoply of hygienic and esthetic procedures (manicure/pedicure, body waxing, hair straightening, makeup, perfume, and dress) that women adopt before a date, a party, or other public events. The idea is not of aligning the body with a preexistent real self. It is about making—*producing*—a body in a rather distinct way. This production of bodies through intervention is not perceived as a threat to the domain of nature in the way that they are shown to be for Europeans and North Americans confronted with new biotechnological developments or in ethical debates over medical enhancement (Edmonds 2010). Although gender is seen to be rooted in natural sexual difference, it is understood that this "nature" is readily alterable. The constant reiteration (whether discursive or material) of sexual difference can be read as a means of consolidating and reenacting this precarious "nature." Rohden (2001, 203) makes this point in her analysis of early twentieth-century Brazilian medical theses on the question of sexual difference: "Doctors [in this period] constantly reiterate that there exists, *de facto* a natural difference between men and women. But this does not mean that it is static or given *a priori*. This difference appears to be subject to external interventions. It is natural, but not definitive. In truth, if it was definitively given by purely biological and immutable variables, the menace on its integrity would not have called these doctors' attention to such a degree" (my translation).

In European anthropology, Strathern (1992b, 53) argues, "culture" was implicitly played off nature: "A sense of change was seen against a sense of constraint, future possibility against what was assumed to be given." Speaking of the impact of new reproductive technologies such as IVF for the notion of nature, Strathern remarked on the late-twentieth-century perception of a natural world ever more subject to artificial management. The development of new technical means of intervening into lived vitality raised questions for the way the relation between what was taken to be "immutable in social life" and "what is open to change and innovation" (53) was being reconfigured. Strathern shows how, as the grounding provided by nature—its incontrovertibility—was (conceptually) eroded, increasing importance was given to choice in the "enterprising" culture. This both opened up possibilities and gave rise to the uncomfortable sentiment that the realm of nature was shrinking under the onslaught of human artifice. Twenty-five years on, the recursive analogical interplay between the domains of nature and artifice holds strong. Franklin (2014, 9) notes that Strathern (1992), like Rabinow (1996), predicted that once the grounding function of nature had disappeared, the analogic flow would be interrupted and nature would cease to provide the merographic operator or analogic model for culture. Drawing on her work on how biology itself has become a technology (such as when stem cells become "tools"), Franklin (2014, 13) argues that the potential for merographic connection has not been lost but that the analogy travels back: "It may be that as a newly biologized and technologized nature has morphed into instrumentalized biology . . . the grounding function of nature has not disappeared but is simply performing a traditional symbolic function." This enterprising up of the biological has given rise—through what Franklin calls "analogic return"—to a more contingent and relative understanding of what biology is. Nature, Franklin argues, "is a less 'original' condition than are the historically acquired norms often modelled upon it" (14), while not becoming entirely dissociated from the idea that it is more solid or prior to sociality. Interestingly, Franklin notes, a commonsense determination refuses to understand "nature" or "biology" as entirely contingent. "We see examples of this tendency to reify and essentialize all the time—in the classroom, in the newspapers, and in the scholarly literature" (14). Helmreich (2011) points to a similar tension in an article entitled "What Was Life?," where he traces the way biotechnologies are unwinding the facts of life, destabilizing their naturalistic foundations and moving them from the domain of the given to that of the contingent. This undoing of the self-evidence of what "life" is has placed us in an ambiguous relation and enduring pursuit of the natural. "In the bargain, 'nature' becomes everywhere and nowhere, both completely given and thoroughly constructed" (683). The tension between continuity and change that much of the scholarship on health and the new biotechnologies traces is often presented as a novelty or as a paradox that needs to be accounted for. In the remainder of this discussion I draw on the work of anthropologist Mattijs van de Port (2011, 2012), who proposes to read Bahia through the lens of "the baroque," and return to philosopher Catherine Malabou's notion of plasticity to attempt to speak to this tension between biological contingency, technological possibility, and the sense of loss that it often entails. As we saw at the outset of this book, *plasticity*, from the Greek *plassein*, refers to the capacity to both give *and* receive form. For Malabou, the conceptual and political promise of "plasticity" resides precisely in this amplitude of meaning. Yet, she notes insistently, metaphors of fixity or rigidity continue to abide and prevail over ones of malleability. "Why do we ignore our own plasticity?," she wonders repeatedly. In many ways this conundrum matches the one I have been tracing here regarding the tenaciousness of the idea of the bounded body. What makes the reification so enduring?

In a highly evocative passage in which she describes her father's death, Haraway (2008, 162–63) illuminates some of what is at stake in the reification of the body: "To come to accept the body's unmaking, I need to remember its becoming." Remembering the moment when her father's presence in his body dulled, she writes: "No, as his body cooled, his *body* was no longer there. The corpse is not the body. Rather, the body is always in the making; it is a vital entanglement of heterogeneous scales, times, and kinds of beings webbed into fleshy presence, always a becoming, always constituted in relating" (162–63).

To evoke this powerful moment of her father's body's undoing is to point to the existential stakes in the work of holding bodies together. These perpetual "un/doings" of lived bodies show up a dark other side to bodily plasticity: death. For only a dead body is no longer plastic, Haraway powerfully reminds us.[2]

*Every*body Is Plastic (or the Problem of Comparison)

Van de Port (2012) also found that the natural is not, in his words, the only anchor ground for "the real" in Salvador. Bahians, he proposes, wholeheartedly opt for that which is evidently fabricated and undeniably made up: "'The natural' is not constantly mobilized to upgrade the reality calibre of cultural constructions" (872). Artifice does not make something less real, or diminish its appeal, quite the contrary. This positions desire at the center of (what he refers to as) "the real." The stable, grounded, incontestable nature of "the real of desire," as he refers to it, is particularly powerful in worlds where certainties are lost and where the power of the natural referent is absent (878). Van de Port's insight has a double importance because it provides a theoretical bridge between two otherwise unrelated sets of ethnographic observations that are repeatedly made regarding Salvador, namely the absence of the reference of the natural and the coexistence of sensuality, joy, and violence. As such it accounts for the peculiar libidinous economy that sustains and nourishes desires for ever-expanding realms of intervention and enhancements. In his monograph *Ecstatic Encounters*, van de Port (2011, 173–74) argues that this "unremitting self-instruction that 'reality is artifice'" is precisely what sustains the cravings for "a reconciliation with nature."

However, he argues that the anthropologist (him)self does not escape the constructivist double bind: "the anthropologist's statement that what is presented as 'natural' is in fact a social construct does not temper his desire for exactly this 'natural' that has been dismissed as fake." While I find his analysis of Bahian sociality incredibly evocative and important, I wonder to what extent the critique he levels at anthropology that to bring flesh and body into textual analysis is an "unstated project of bringing 'nature' and 'essence' back into academic world depictions" or to succumb to an urge to soil the conventions of academia with body fluids, excrement, and carnal activities (van de Port 2011, 175) does not reproduce the constructive deadlock it seeks to evade. In an intriguing passage in which he mobilizes Aretxaga and Kristeva, van de Port argues that bodies and their effusions—as overdetermined primordial symbols—are never reducible to cultural analysis, no matter how sophisticated (176). The problem, I would argue, is that van de Port is speaking of the work that "evocations" of the carnal and visceral do in a text. Evocations are necessarily strategic and partial and therefore relate primarily to discursive practices. They are the stuff of the "Grand Theory" he seeks to destabilize through them. I have attempted to situate my analysis of bodies in a radically different analytical frame. In attending to the myriad differences that are produced through quotidian bodily practices, such as those around the management of menstrual bleeding or hormone use, we can begin to reduce the gap that van de Port laments holds us from ever accessing "the Real." We can begin to construct texts that do not begin with assumptions about where the Real is (often, implicitly, in "Nature") and where excess ("Culture") lies.

Van de Port (2011, 39) reads the Bahian esthetic preference for the artificial through the lens of the Baroque, the spirit of which he found to be omnipresent in Bahia. Baroque and classic esthetics are artfully counterposed in his analysis. He shows that the classic esthetics that are the preferred style of academic knowledge production foreground "a morphology of—and concomitant preference for—*fixed forms*, delineation, clarity, order, categorical purity" (35), whereas baroque aesthetics trouble categories, drawing attention to "the lack that is at the heart of all totalizing narratives" (37): "the inclination is to move towards the fusion and mingling of opposites, towards connectivity, towards an elasticity and fluidity that allows for absorption and encompassment. Bahia wants you to be dazzled, rather than sharp-eyed" (62). Baroque forms flourished in worlds "where people found themselves caught betwixt-and-between irreconcilable paradigms and enmeshed in violent social and political upheaval" (van de Port 2012, 879). Bahia, with its heritage of slavery and the omnipresence of violence, is marked by a collective trauma that, van de Port suggests, feeds the spirit of baroque. This is because trauma, through the ruptures it brings about, reveals that the moral and social order that are otherwise taken for granted are "founded on make-belief" (879). We can read van de Port diffractively through the feminist trope of analogical return (Franklin 2014) to question what happens when the natural referent disappears, when its metaphorical nature is made apparent. What van de Port's ethnographically situated reading makes vividly apparent is the tremendous prolificity of desire and excess that is unleashed—and which ethnographers of Brazil struggle to account for within the classic Marxian frame—when the scope of intervention is not fully capped by reference to what is naturally given. Highlighting falsity generates unstaunchable desire, in sum.

Because the polarity that van de Port sets up between the baroque and the classical is situated at one end (the baroque one) in Bahia, it makes it seem as though the classic also has a specific locality (the locus of academic knowledge-making, often short-handed as "Western").[3] In attempting to account for the specificities that mark the places we describe, we as anthropologists are often still plagued by the idea of a situatedness of difference, as something pertaining to a locality or culture. This is very much a product of the discursive practices of setting up comparisons—implicit or explicit. The question then becomes how much we attribute to the place in the description and how we construct it as "a place." This reveals a specific difficulty pertaining to writing anthropologically of urban Brazil with which I have also grappled. Writing about other places—places we are embroiled with in complex ways—often serves the function of decentering the place from which we write (which, regardless of where "we" are from, carries through academic conventions the remnants of tenacious dualisms). This leads me to the difficult terrain of situating myself more explicitly. Having benefited from the freedom and placelessness that come from migrations several generations deep, a multilingual upbringing and having myself grown up between Europe and North and South America—not to mention secondhand experience of the topic at hand as the daughter of an anthropologist and a doctor—I sought to locate myself in a place that felt neither exotic nor quite home (wherever that could have been). My project was to study biomedical practices ethnographically. That I sought to study biomedicine in Brazil was not a deliberate attempt to exoticize it. It was motivated by a desire to do symmetrical anthropology, and open up to ethnographic inquiry the practice of biomedicine. I opted to do this in Bahia, fueled by a mixture of serendipity, linguistic convenience, curiosity, and in an effort to decenter the universal associations that the practice of biomedicine might hold. This has run me into difficult waters, for I have done so while attempting all the while to eschew a portrayal of Bahian biomedical practices as an incomplete or imperfect version of a proper biomedicine, as practiced in some professedly global center. The anthropology of science, Viveiros de Castro and Goldman (2012, 425) argue, has had an important impact on anthropological theory writ large: It has served to erode the Great Divisions (science/nonscience, modern/nonmodern, humans/nonhumans, and so on) on which Western modernity's devices of subjectivation were (and to some extent continue to be) founded. Such a device is at work in the vexed question—for many members of the traditional middle and upper classes—of Brazil's incomplete modernity, development, and general "place" in the world, or in the tenacious idea that Brazil is somehow still catching up.[4] It permeates debates concerning cultural change and multiple modernities in Brazil. For example, Darcy Ribeiro (1995) notes that "we" (Brazilians) have internalized the idea of being incompletely civilized, non-European, and yet have no clear identification with another (internal) culture, having decimated indigenous cultures and coexisted with African culture solely through enslavement. The terms *hybridity* and *syncretism* are brought in to explain the coexistence of different bodily ontologies or models of healing. But such terms assume distinctly bounded cultural entities and do little to account for how they relate. How, then, to write ethnographically about such processes? Or as Viveiros de Castro and Goldman (2012) put it, where and who are "we" and to what goals do we do ethnographic work? This has been an endlessly difficult question for me as I engage in the task of writing ethnographic theory through Bahia and from a place that—given my own history and origins—continues to shift.[5] On the basis of my experience of living and unraveling my thinking about bodies in Bahia, I have come to feel that the understandings I have produced out of Bahia pertain less to it in some kind of ontological sense than to a reading of bodies through a Bahian lens. Like van de Port, my fieldnotes are replete with quandaries over the limits of the linguistic and conceptual categories I brought with me to the field, and my dazzled response to the vibrant and often violent limitless possibilities that noncontradictoriness enables. My encounter with Bahia and with questions pertaining to bodies taught me less about Bahian bodies than it did about the problems of translation that come with the experience of displacement.[6] In drawing on critical feminist theory (Barad 2007; Grosz 1994; Haraway 1991, 1992, 1997, 2008; Kristeva 1982; Mol 2002); history of science and medicine (Duden 1991; Fausto-Sterling 2000; Laqueur 1990; Oudshoorn 1994); or the work of Melanesian ethnographers (Strathern 1988, 1991, 1992a, 1992b; Weiner 1995), my aim has been to reveal that bodies are made stable, unitary, or fixed only through the practices that enact them as such or through the academic conventions that have rendered the abstraction "the body" ontological. In this sense, I am not arguing that Bahian bodies are plastic—as opposed to purported "Western" bodies—but that everybody is plastic.

That I argue this with ethnographic materials concerning biomedical practices in Bahia should not be read as implying that the plastic quality of bodies is somehow greater there than it might be elsewhere. At most, I hope this text be read as implying that Bahians are less delusional about this fact than other people perhaps are. It is easier to recognize bodily plasticity from Bahia, as it were. The need to resist the localizing, essentializing, and Othering tendencies that get read into the comparisons we draw up is a move to resist a classical mode of world making that produces questions about how "heres" and "theres" relate, or about where particular cultural forms (animist, totemic, naturalist, analogic, perspectivist, and so on) reside. The problem is that in alluding to the difference, the alterity, of other forms of world making, we remain tied to a dialectic of difference that (re)produces the problem it tries to evade. This particular issue has a long history in Brazil. It can be traced back to poet Oswald de Andrade's 1928 *Manifesto antropófago* (Anthropophage Manifesto). Andrade rewrites chronology, claiming

1928 as the year 374 since the swallowing of the Portuguese Bishop Sardinha, who was devoured by Indians in the sixteenth century, an episode that Andrade playfully suggests should be considered the founding moment of Brazil (year 1). *Antropófagia* inverses — or resymmetricizes — the relation between Brazil and Europe, inverting the extractivist trope of absorbing the vitality of the Other. It is a striking metaphor of postcolonial relations. It speaks to the questions Brazilian elites were already posing nearly a century ago regarding their relation to "universal" (read: European) esthetics and values on the one hand and — as elites — to the internal Others that make up Brazilian diversity.[7] In an essay on the divine cannibalism of the Araweté — a variation of Tupi cannibalism that inspired Andrade — Eduardo Viveiros de Castro (2007b) argues that what is assimilated in such ritual forms is the position of the devoured: his condition as an enemy. The Anthropophage Manifesto, in this reading, enables the postcolonial devourer to exchange positions with the colonizer. The full implications of Viveiros de Castro's rereading of the Manifesto's decolonizing potential have yet to be released. It is a tool that (along with others) may hold the potential for further decolonizing anthropological theory. This is a highly idiosyncratic manner of perturbing modernist categories: not by confronting them with an alternative system (the Melanesian dividual, Asian hot/cold systems, African hematological classifications, and so on) but by devouring them. For Viveiros de Castro (2007a, 129), antropófagia is "a weapon to fight the cultural subjectivation of Latin America, Indians and non-Indians alike, by European and Christian paradigms" (my translation).

Therefore, to evoke the plasticity of bodies *from* Bahia (rather than *in* Bahia) is to attend to the conditions under which bodies are discursively held together — or not — as fixed and bounded entities. As I have tried to show through the ethnography, the way that the materiality of bodies matters in Salvador is specific. The most pervasive set of answers I was given about the specificity of Bahian modes of embodiment concerned the fact that, there, bodies are more exposed, closer to the surface of public exchange. Their transformations are the object of very public collective evaluations. In speaking about what seemed to be a shared observation that bodies occupied a prominent public place in Bahian sociality, my *Soteropolitanos* friends or informants almost systematically alluded to climate. What was odd to them was the absence of the body in Europe, which they repeatedly associated with its disappearance under layers of protective clothing. Thus bundled up, removed from the everyday, bodies surely must fester and recede from presence. It is no wonder, I was told again and again, that the French developed reason against the senses, against the body, wrapped up as they were in all that clothing, removed as they were from their bodies' sensations. One dear friend who had lived in Paris for several years recalled with a unique physicality to her language the extraordinary collective experience of peeling off layers of clothing after a long hard winter, the liberation of bodies from the layers of cloth, the incredible—in her words—sensual energy that permeated the spring as the sun and air touched upon bodies that had been enclosed for so long, hidden from experience. In Bahia, the social work that must be invested in making bodies is made particularly visible, in ways I have attempted to render through ethnography. My point, then, is not that bodies elsewhere are not also made but that discursive and symbolic practices attempt more to conceal or naturalize this work. The materialities of bodies in Bahia intra-act with specific historical contingencies, institutional configurations, to produce specific local epistemologies of bodily becomings. These specific, local, bodily intra-actions render bodies knowable in particular ways. They produce fleshy differences.

From Inseparability to Resistance: On the Politics of *L'écart*

In the final section I return to the notion of plasticity that Malabou has developed to dwell on the possibilities it affords as a locus of an ethics of care. Malabou proposes that plasticity offers a semantic resistance to the notion of flexibility that has been so heavily invested by neoliberalism. In the preface to the 2011 French re-edition of *Que Faire de Notre Cerveau*, Malabou repositions plasticity as a "weapon," as the resistance that form offers to flexibility. This resistance, she proposes, can be deployed against capital, from *within* the dynamic of power as opposed to outside it. Drawing inspiration from Foucault's insight that resistance to power cannot be external to its capillarities, Malabou (2011, 25) proposes that the concept of plasticity—given its twin poles of continuity and change, contingency and possibility—offers a unique *internal* resistance. Through the conceptual possibilities afforded by plasticity she hopes to elaborate a biopolitical theory that moves beyond the opposition (or écart) between the biological and the symbolic. In her words, plasticity does not describe a signifying economy that can be separated from its material base: "Plasticity is not, like sexuality for Foucault, difference for Derrida or multiplicity for Deleuze the floating signifier, the surplus or the gap [*case vide*] that enables a mobile reordering of the real" (26, my translation).[8] She suggests that the persistence of the écart between meaning and matter, structure and content, symbolic and biological, at the heart of political philosophy is the reason for which critique cannot escape its assimilation by capital. In her words: "The symbolic supplement is the theoretical equivalent to profit" (26–27, my translation). This écart that separates the symbolic and the material is precisely where she locates, after Boltanski and Chiapello (1999), the replicative power of capital and its capacity to ingest and absorb critique.

This is perhaps the point at which Malabou's hopefulness is at its most fragile. It is the point on which she has received strongest critique. She articulates her political theory of plasticity around the fact that, in her reading, neurobiology has rendered the symbolic and material plasticity of the brain indistinguishable from each other. Her work on the neuroplasticity of the brain challenged her, she tells us, to develop a new theory of meaning (du sens)[9] that does not break with matter. That is, she hopes to draw out from neurobiology a political philosophy that is not founded on the écart, on the break between the symbolic and the biological. To Žižek (2006, 26), who has argued that "the status of the Real is purely parallactic and, as such, non-substantial: it has no substantial density in itself, it is just a gap between two points of perspective, perceptible only in the shift from the one to the other,"[10] she asks, "what if there was no écart at all?" (Malabou 2011, 29, my translation). To make the claim that neurobiology shows matter and consciousness to be inseparable and continuous, Malabou relies largely on what Fitzgerald and Callard (2014) describe as a select reading of neurobiologists' popular science or "cross-over" publications for lay audiences. They describe Malabou's engagement with the neurosciences as "ebullient." This form of engagement, in their view, takes the statements of the neuroscience as true without attending to the fierce epistemological or ontological debates that mark these sciences. While her cultural theory is astute and thorough, they lament that it is based on a reading of the neuroscientific fact that is surprisingly thin. Clearly, Malabou is not a science and technology studies (STS) scholar and as such does not concern herself with the politics of fact building. This is an important shortcoming that in the end disserves her, as it forecloses "the space for a dynamic and mutually constitutive traffic" (Fitzgerald and Callard 2014) across biology and culture. It produces its own unwitting écarts, between matters of fact and matters of concern, to return to a well-trodden distinction (Latour 2004). Likewise, Leys (2011) expresses concerns over Malabou's use of neurobiology and reads her as naturalizing contemporary politics and culture. She argues that authors such as Damasio and LeDoux, on whom Malabou almost entirely depends in her analysis, are "mistaken" in their subordination of the fact of plasticity to the notion of flexible adaptation and biological survival. "Above all, they have obfuscated the difficulty of theorizing the transition from the neuronal to the mental," she remarks (Leys 2011), thus challenging any claim Malabou makes regarding neurobiology's potential to move us beyond the opposition (or écart) between the biological and the symbolic.

While I am in no place to argue for the veracity of the claims she makes through neurobiology, and largely agree with these critical readings regarding Malabou's surprisingly uncritical mobilization of biological facts, I find the notion of plasticity that she defends incredibly important. Its conceptual value does not entirely depend on the veracity of the biological facts out of which it is constructed. Further, it is a notion that can be extended beyond the brain-organ to the whole body, as I have done here.[11] Her theoretical redeployment of plasticity provides an important resource for feminist-inflected STS analyses of the shifting relations between the material and the cultural. Plasticity's forcefulness as a concept resides first and foremost in the way that it holds together a contradiction: "between the maintenance of the system, or 'homeostasis,' and the ability to change the system or 'self-generation'" (Malabou 2011, 173, my translation). This is another means of conceptualizing the analogical traffic between continuity and change, between nature and artifice, between biology and culture. It is yet another way to frame the question of intra-action, agential realism, or entanglement (Barad 2007), fleshy infoldings (Haraway 2008, 249), material semiotics (Haraway 1991), transcorporeality, or meeting-with-matter (see Hird 2009 for a critical review of feminist engagements with matter). It brings these poles within a common conceptual space, while calling attention to the explosiveness that their friction entails. This seems all the more important at a time when the social sciences are becoming acutely more aware of the problems that the boundaries produced out of the inherited binaries that occupy our models set up to our understanding the world in which we live. Whether it is ontologically more complex and enmeshed than it was before is a question for the historians, but in the wake of the growing scholarship on the Anthropocene (Bonneuil and Fressoz 2013; Stengers 2014) and attention to intraspecies entanglements (Abrahamsson and Bertoni 2014; Haraway 2008; Kirksey 2014) or to complex scalar relations at work in epigenetics (Landecker and Panofsky 2013), it is clear that we need a range of models that can hold together the binaries while pointing to their constitutive force. What I am trying to articulate here, after Malabou, is the tremendous energy (both productive and destructive) that these constitutive tensions generate.

Explosive Choices: From Matters of Fact to Matters of *Care*

Plasticity, then, should not be read as a eulogy to a promissory regime of self-optimization. I hope to have made clear throughout this book that "self"-transformation is seldom about the self in Bahia and that it does not operate against the primacy of a given natural body. What I have focused less on in this book, partly because of its conspicuous absence from public discourse (despite my questions in this direction), is the *cost* of plasticity. Malabou posits a third pole to the concept of plasticity: one that bridges the dialectics between the constancy of form and the transformative potential of plasticity. Identity ("the" Self, in her writing) is the product of a funda-mental tension between homeostasis and self-making (Malabou 2011, 161). But given that plasticity is *not* flexibility, mutations leave traces and marks of the resistance that form opposes to transformation: We destroy ourselves a little as we transform ourselves.

This book has focused more on the perceived emancipatory side of plas-ticity, emphasizing the way in which, in Bahia, work on and through bodies is seen to have social effects. The dark side of this plasticity, the costs it places on organisms' homeostatic capacities (a process that Illich [1976] referred to as the iatrogenic effects of medicalization), the corrosiveness of chemical regimes of living, and the potential explosiveness of subsequent pilings-on of interventions have been less at the center of this narrative. This is not because I am not concerned by them, but rather because the explo-siveness of choices is downplayed, outright denied, or set into risk–benefit analyses that, in characteristically forward-looking Brazilian fashion, focus on the potential opened by intervention and less on the losses this may entail.[12] The relative absence of the dark side of plasticity in this narrative is also the product of an ethnographic concern with situating bodily plas-ticity—diffracted through the Bahian practices I describe here—in a frame that does not mourn for the "natural" or the unintervened body. Underscor-ing this oftentimes implicit view is the ideal of a return to pure matters of fact, to material contingencies, that I do not believe are reliable grounds to articulate a feminist critique from, given their sticky, embroiled, and messy nature.

In a context where interventions are widespread, the idea of the "natural" itself is intervened with. In the vernacular form, intervention nevertheless pertains to a lexicon that is—along with technology or artifice—usually set against "nature." In this work I have been carving out a different use for the term, one that does not assume that interventions necessarily breach limits. The term *intervention*—from the Latin for "to come between"—carries the idea of the delimitations that bound the thing into which interventions are carried out. My suggestion has been that interventions do not breach (pre)bounded entities but rather contribute to constituting them as bounded. In Euro-American knowledge practices, emphasis is often placed on the end product of this transformation (the bounded entity), concealing the practices that enact a thing as a delimited whole. This makes the boundaries of the myriad enacted wholes appear fairly self-evident and fixed, a point that Mol (2002) made most eloquently. I do not mean to imply that all biomedical interventions are equal or that it is not possible to adopt—in function of context—criteria from which to differentiate, or indeed prioritize, certain interventions from others. My point has been simply to suggest that the distinction "not intervened in"/"intervened in" (read: natural/cultural) is not the correct site to evaluate the politics of intervention. The unfurling development of biomedical interventions has raised the question of choice in a new way as the distinction between treating injury, or remedying illness, and enhancement becomes increasingly difficult to make. Many commentators in Brazil worry that choices concerning biomedical interventions such as elective cesarean births, plastic surgery, or menstrual suppression are essentially market-driven. The exhortation to choose the normal is founded, as Pottage (1998) showed, on a tautological rationale. Elaborating on the implications of Canguilhem's model of norms, according to which although the abnormal is logically secondary to the normal, Pottage notes that it is existentially prior to practices of normalization. The normal—as defined contextually—is the outcome of an ongoing normative project that continuously transforms the understanding and perception of normality (Pottage 1998, 12; see also Hacking 2007). The concern this gives rise to is that interventions are seen as potentially infinite—themselves limitless—as the idea of normality itself shifts. Choosing, as Strathern (1992b, 37) notes, is in such contexts no longer a matter of choice: "The enterprising self . . . is not just one who is able to choose between alternative ways, but one who implements that choice through consumption (self-enhancement) and for whom there is, in a sense, no choice not to consume. . . . The sense that one has no choice not to consume is a version of the feeling that one has no choice not to make a choice. Choice is imagined as the only source of difference: this is the collapsing effect of the market analogy."

It is particularly helpful to think about the ways in which women are now being exhorted to "choose when to menstruate," as one widely circulating Association of Reproductive Health Practitioners slogan goes. What is striking about the menstrual suppression debate is the remarkable absence of a discussion of potential health risks. This is despite the fact that—where the extended-regime pill is concerned—users consume 30 percent more steroid hormones than if they take a monthly interval. Choice is very much the idiom that prevailed in the bizarre combination of *machista* and neofeminist rhetoric that characterizes Coutinho's defense of women's rights. During my last meeting with him, on the eve of departure, he asked me what I thought of menstrual suppression and whether I would be traveling home "free of menstruation." We were on the threshold of his *consultório* in the old center; I was in an emotional whirlwind, preparing to depart from Salvador, in the midst of good-byes. Outside it was raining torrentially. Taken aback by his nevertheless characteristic move to resituate me as patient, as woman, as menstruator, I answered that for many of the women I had interviewed menstrual suppression brought about a relief from menstrual cramps or premenstrual tension, but that it was not something I would consider for myself. He laughed and, stroking my cheek, paternalistically exclaimed, "See, woman is free to choose, *filha* [daughter], if you *gosta* [enjoy] menstruating, *fica a vontade* [do as you please/be my guest]! But I know one thing, the more women know about the possibility of not menstruating, the more they will choose to free themselves of her [menstruation]."

Needless to say, this commentary left me feeling very ambiguous about what response one could give, what the implications of writing—as an intervention—might be. What Coutinho articulated with staggering clarity was what Boltanski and Chiapello (1999) describe in their *Spirit of Capitalism*. Coutinho seemed to be saying to me, "all news is good news," or that no matter what critique I might articulate, it would be subsumed by the logic of choice. A key insight I draw from van de Port's or Taussig's Lacanian readings of the way violence and desire cohabit in Latin America is that this logic of choice is embroiled in an apparently limitless spiral that simultaneously produces desire for more intervention and more nature. This is how we can read the chemically (hormonally) assisted return to a purportedly natural amenorrheic body.

Given this plasticity, given its inherent internal tension and potentially "explosive" or costly impact, how should "the good" of bodily interventions be assessed? I hope to have convinced the reader that plasticity is not a prescriptive idea (that is, I am not suggesting that bodies should be intervened in) but is rather mobilized here in a descriptive or interpretative mode. Given the plasticity that I have read into bodies, what ethics are we to defend? This book has suggested that ethical, rights-based evaluations concerning bodily interventions often center on ideas of a bounded, autonomous body. While I have sought to problematize this notion, I do not believe that all interventions are equal. One issue in this debate is the somewhat teleological assumptions that at times underscore the idea of bodily intervention, enhancement, or optimization as a project, with an end point, or goal (be this one of health, amelioration, or restoration). As I have tried to demonstrate, bodily interventions are almost always accompanied by such rhetorical strategies. These force their evaluation into risk–benefit-type analyses with choice outcomes. But what if we supplant the notion of project with that of *design*, as Latour (2011), after Sloterdijk, suggests we do? How might the notion of design open up different forms of ethical evaluations for our chemical infoldings and fleshy entanglements with technologies? Latour proposes that Sloterdijk's concept of design enables a move out of modernist concerns with objects, into the realm of *things*. Things, as we saw, unlike objects, come enmeshed in what Latour terms matters of concern (contra matters of fact). They are gatherings. As such, design (versus object making) is by definition a collaborative endeavor: "even if in some cases the 'collaborators' are not all visible, welcomed or willing" (Latour 2011, 156). Drawing on this we can say that the ethical question is no longer *should we design?* (given that design permeates all human and nonhuman endeavors) but *how do we design?* Design, in short, necessarily has an ethical dimension, but this ethical dimension is not one that can be traced back to matters of fact.

To conclude, then, I have suggested that Malabou's genealogical development of the concept of plasticity be added to the repertoire of theoretical engagements with the comings-into-being of form and matter. This concept brings with it a critical attention to the way in which the intertwinement of continuity and change rests on a delicate balance that has potentially explosive effects. We need to learn to live with the explosive, and potentially corrosive, character of plasticity, without yearning for a lost stable referent or investing too much hope in an endlessly flexible promissory future. This implies deciding collectively what costs are acceptable (which relies on having the conditions to make these known). Critique can play a role in showing up what human or organic (for want of a better term) costs are being concealed, strategically rendered uncertain, or deliberately ignored. But it cannot rely on matters of fact. I am often deeply uncomfortable with the naturalizing tendencies of much of the ecofeminist critique that has been most vocal about menstrual suppression. Yet I also find the promissory technology-confident antithesis to it naïve and oblivious to the exclusions or power dynamics at work in the stratified worlds in which these technological hopes are dreamed. In this sense, we may need to move the entire discussion to *matters of care*—envisioned as an entangled ethicopolitical issue (de la Bellacasa 2011). Matters of care are thicker than the politics of matters of concern, they add to concern an engagement in their becomings (100). If, as I have argued, entities don't preexist the work of relating them, the relations we build between them have consequences. One consequence I hope may flow from this is the demonstration of the potential for deflagration that is ignited out of Malabou's holding together of the twin poles of plasticity. If anything, it adds an important conceptual tool to a critical aspect of *caring* that feminist scholarship has done much to reveal, namely that caring is also a practice of refusing purity and highlighting the "dirty" (Haraway 1997, 36), messy, incomplete, paradoxical, and oftentimes contradictory natures of realities.

NOTES

Introduction: Plastic Bodies

1. See Natansohn (2005) for a detailed analysis of the women's programs on which Coutinho appeared as a gynecologist and on their portrayal of gender relations and women's bodies.

2. The Oxford University Press English edition's title is more subdued than the Portuguese original, which would translate as "Menstruation: Useless Bleeding."

3. Ninety percent of the press articles presenting menstrual suppression (from *Cosmopolitan* to *Time* or the *Washington Post*) present the arguments put forward by Coutinho and Segal in *Is Menstruation Obsolete?* (Johnston-Robledo, Barnack, and Wares 2006). Advocates of menstrual suppression are quoted twice as often as opponents, thus biasing coverage and massively downplaying potential risks or uncertainties that prevail around the practice.

4. For a detailed review of the new hormonal contraceptives currently being developed, see Bahamondes and Bahamondes (2014).

5. These rates are highly variable internationally, as a Population Reference Bureau (Clifton, Kaneda, and Ashford 2008) analysis reveals. Worldwide, only 8 percent of married women use the pill, although this represents more than 3.5 billion people. The rate is 18 percent for "more developed" nations and reaches 45 percent in France, which has one of the highest national rates. Four percent of the world's married women use hormonal injections, with particularly high rates in South Africa (28 percent) and Malawi (30 percent).

6. It found its rationale in the limited uptake of the pill worldwide, a fact that was accounted for by reference to the heterogeneity of women's personal, cultural, and religious circumstances.

7. Online source; no page numbers.

8. The literature on the safety of extended-regime oral contraceptives and long-acting hormonal methods principally comprises epidemiological studies that tend to downplay risks (e.g., Edelman et al. 2014; Isley and Kaunitz 2011) and feminist analyses that alert to the fact that these drugs are often used without adequate evaluations of their potential health risks (e.g., Corrêa 1998; Mintzes, Hardon, and Hanhart 1993).

9. The classification of combined oral contraceptives relies on the progestins used. The first and second generation include norethisterone and levonorgestrel; the third and fourth include gestodene (e.g., Arianna, Careza, Meliane) and drospirenone (e.g., Yasmin, Yasminelle 28, Yaz, Aliane).

10. Some articles relativize such increased risks, noting that "the additional risk of thrombosis with a 3rd vs. 2nd generation pill would be ... —at worst—one more death in a million users" (DeLoughery 2011). Likewise, Spitzer (1997) concluded that the relative risk of thrombosis is real but "clinically unimportant and of no public health significance." Such minor risks can become potentially massive public crises, however, as we saw in the UK pill crisis of 1995 and more recently in France. Mylène Rouzaud-Cornabas is currently completing a project on the anatomy of this recent crisis, and I thank her for her input here. Controversy over the potential cancer-preventing or cancer-inducing effects of these drugs also marked the fields of contraceptive and hormone replacement therapy. A recent review suggested that none of the large, prospective cohort studies have observed an increased overall risk of cancer incidence among ever-users of oral contraceptives; indeed, several have suggested important long-term benefits, such as reduced endometrial cancer risk of 50 percent among ever-users (Cibula et al. 2010). This review was followed by a letter to the editor alerting to the skewness of the data presented, to which the authors declined to respond. There is remarkably little in the literature on how the debate is structured by possible conflicts of interest or how ignorance and absences in the existent knowledge on potential risks are actively produced (McGoey 2012; Proctor and Schiebinger 2008), with the notable exception of Löwy's (2012, 2013) work. The Committee on Women, Population, and the Environment released a Depo-Provera Fact Sheet in 2007 in which they ascertain that in papers filed with the U.S. Securities and Exchange Commission, Upjohn admitted that, in order to secure sales of Depo-Provera abroad, it made payments of more than $4 million to employees of foreign governments from 1971 to 1975. http://cwpe.org/node/185, accessed January 23, 2015.

11. In a heavily biased article, Isley and Kaunitz (2011) argue that the advantages of Depo-Provera far outweigh what they refer to as "theoretical" health concerns with bone mineral density and conclude that these should not "restrict initiation or continuation."

12. All of which were performed in less time than a single tubal ligation, under local anesthetic, while doctor and patient exchanged jokes.

13. Christianity plays a central role in the way Bahians think about reproduction, and the body more generally. I have often been questioned about how the things I describe coexist with what is rightly seen as a heavily religious context. However, such questions are based on a more or less explicit assumption of the incoherence between Christian belief on the one hand and contraceptive practice on the other, which is seldom experienced as contradiction or incoherence by the women I met.

14. The private or "supplementary" sector is defined as that which is not financed through the Ministry of Health. In practice, however, supplementary medicine often receives state funding. It is heterogeneous and funded through a range of different organizations, which include health insurance (provided by general or specialized insurance companies) and a plethora of medical groups and cooperatives that often have their own structures (hospitals, practices, etc.) or contract services through an elaborate system of conventions. Patients contract medical insurance either through their employer or privately. According to the 1990 IBGE census, of the 362 medical establishments in Salvador, 246 were private (cited in da Silva et al. 1997). Of these 246 institutions, 86 percent of these were for profit and 12 percent philanthropic, and only 51 percent of these institutions were completely independent of public funding. These are for the majority small units, consisting of four or fewer consultórios, and the most frequently offered specialties were gynecology (46 percent) and pediatrics (40 percent) (da Silva et al. 1997).

15. Private insurance varies widely in price, with the lowest entry plans at under US$50 and high-end plans exceeding US$400/month (where the minimum monthly wage is US$292). According to widely circulated figures, a doctor receives less than US$4 per consultation in the SUS, and according to several doctors I spoke with, a private consultation earns them on average US$10 (although the consultation can cost as much as US$200). In recent years, Salvador has seen an increase in "popular clinics," which are not linked to the SUS or to the system planos, and offer consultations and diagnostic services at a reduced cost. These tend to be located in popular neighborhoods on the periphery or in the old center. Gynecological consultation and Pap tests figure highly among the services sought from these clinics, where patients are more rapidly served than in the SUS, and prices are cheaper than in private clinics, as money is transferred directly between doctor and patient, rather than through the system of planos. As intermediaries between state and private health institutions, these institutions increase the complexity of the health provision landscape in a context where the consumption of health services and adherence to a plano are constantly renegotiated as a function of needs, priorities, and changing circumstances.

16. These effectively returned women's health to a focus on the mother–child dyad, which focuses on women exclusively as mothers and which Diniz characterizes as a "sexist and authoritarian system of medical practice"—at the expense of a genuine sexual and reproductive health policy. Part of the problem is that the health professionals in the SUS are mistrained and unprepared for primary care (Aquino 2014), and that the training of midwives to take increased responsibility for women's health continues to be strongly opposed by the medical establishment (Diniz 2012). Despite huge

improvements in access to health care, women's health indicators (such as severe maternal morbidity, which is four times higher than in developed countries) are "embarrassing for Brazil," threatening the notion that "the more intervention the better" (Diniz 2012, 127).

17. In 2000, over 60 percent of the population had completed only primary education and only 8 percent entered into some kind of higher-education degree program requiring the completion of secondary education (Figoli 2006). Given these stark differences, education levels give a fairly good idea of social differences. Mello and Novais (1998) state that the number of employees with a *carteira assinada* (formal contract) grew eightfold, from 3 million in 1960 to 23.8 million in 1980. In the period 1970–1980, female employment in Brazil grew by 92 percent.

18. There is a long debate within Brazilian social theory concerning the relative importance of class and race in the making of social hierarchies. Winant (1992, 177) argues that race was often reduced to class, leading racial phenomena to go unrecognized. This argument is made in favor of a more adversarial racial politics that names racism clearly. However, Sansone (2003) and Fry (2000) have argued that this is a form of Eurocentrism that maps an essentially North American vision of race onto the Brazilian context, without considering the numerous intermediary racial categorizations that prevail in Brazil, or their highly relational and subjective character. In naming the social hierarchies I encountered during fieldwork "class" rather than "race" I am not claiming that a transition from race to class has occurred and that race is not a relevant category. Far from it. I attend to these social hierarchies through idioms of class rather than idioms of race because these were the primary terms in which these differences were relayed to me.

19. The Brazilian government prides itself in having brought 35 million people into the middle class in 10 years of Workers Party policies. As many of my friends note, however, this principally involved changing the criteria for what counts as middle class. In 2013, the SAE (Secretary for Strategic Issues) defined the middle class as families living with between US$107 and US$376 (http://www.sae.gov.br/site/?p=17351, accessed February 2, 2015). This means that people earning less than minimum wage (set at US$290/month on January 1, 2015) are considered middle class. The minimum monthly salary is established by the Brazilian Constitution as the minimum wage required to meet basic costs of living such as food, housing, health, education, transport, and leisure. According to Cruz (2014), the Department of Statistics and Socieconomic Studies (DIEESE) estimated that given the average cost of the *cesta básica* (or minimum monthly food ration, currently estimated as retailing at roughly US$100) and the cost of housing, the minimum salary should be just over US$1000 (that is, roughly four times higher than it is at present).

20. Likewise, in her ethnography of in vitro fertilization (IVF) in Ecuador, Roberts (2012) reveals the simultaneous malleability and materiality of local conceptions of race, showing how they become embroiled through IVF to older forms of the biopolitical project of whitening.

21. Historians have shown how delimiting the body was integral to the constitution

of modern subjects in Western societies (Bakhtin 1984; Elias 1994; Foucault 2003; Vigarello 2004). For example, Duden (1991, 17) argued that changing the habits of peasants and women, and their accompanying ideas of purging and bleeding to restore health, involved, for the philanthropic reformers of the eighteenth century, the creation of a new "body" that should not "dissipate itself." Attempting to recapture the experiential body of eighteenth-century women, Duden shows that: "In this cosmos the skin does not close off the body, the inside, against the outside world. In like manner the body itself is also never closed off" (11–12).

22. Differences within what might be glossed as Brazilian bodily ontologies are as significant as those between Brazil and wherever else one might be writing from. Although also located in Brazil, my fieldsite is as far removed from the perspectival worlds described by Amazonian anthropologists (for example, Lagrou 2007; Lima 2005; McCallum 2014; Vilaça 2005; Viveiros de Castro 2012, 2014) as is "Euro-America." In fact, for many people I encountered, the stakes of maintaining this distinction are higher than they are in Europe because in Brazil being identified as indigenous remains stigmatizing.

23. This is to say that there is no pure (or presocial) nature out there that cultures can more or less accurately represent to themselves. Natural facts concerning bodies are contingent on the sociomaterial practices that make them knowable. As such, multiple bodily ontologies coexist in all social settings, and my task here is to describe some of the ways in which this coexistence occurs in Bahia.

24. Brazil has the highest number of metabolic/bariatric surgeons in the world (2,750). They performed 65,000 bariatric surgeries in 2011, which is more than twice the rates of France, and over six times the UK rates, coming second to that of the United States and Canada (Buchwald and Oien 2013).

Chapter 1: Managing the Inside, Out

1. It is difficult to correctly evaluate the proportion of couples who use some version of a rhythm method as a contraceptive method. In practice, *fazer tabela* (charting) tends to consist of an intuitive interpretation of more formalized fertility awareness methods, such as those based on temperature charting, and seldom include any actual daily charting. This method is generally based on the recording of days in the cycle and used to estimate the fertile period, during which condoms are adopted.

2. Several women did feel ovulation; however, the existence of specific technologies to chart the menstrual cycle and identify ovulation attests to the fact that this process is less readily "brought to the surface."

3. The sliding of the uterus from its normal position in the pelvic cavity into the vaginal canal.

4. The class dimension is significant here because there is a certain taboo on speaking about sexuality and menstruation to young women in low-income families. This is the way some public health researchers frame the comparatively high fertility rate among teenage low-income women.

5. This Afro-Brazilian martial art/dance form includes detailed exegeses about the body, blood, strength, and social relations.

6. These are derived from ritual food offerings to the *Orixas* and form part of Bahian cuisine. Acarajé is sold on every street corner in central Salvador. It consists of a ball of bean dough deep fried in palm oil and filled with dried shrimp, chilli, vatapá. Traditionally, acarajé was sold by women as a means of generating income for their initiation into Candomblé. Today this is not always the case, but acarajé vendors retain the traditional *baiana* costume (embroidered white cotton dress, turban, and Orixa beads).

7. Limpeza is often constructed against the idea of the Old World as a dirty place. Jokes abound on the subject of Europeans' (particularly the French) lack of hygiene.

8. This carves out a more figurative usage for the term *cleanse* in English, according to the *Oxford English Dictionary*.

9. These qualifications are meant to reflect everyday popular practices Bahians generically call on, as many of my interviewees related adopting practices of limpeza—whether simply using incense around the home, or going to a religious practitioner to perform a ritual—irrespective of whether they declared themselves religious or not.

10. I was not able to follow this up systematically in other schools, but these comments have a value in their own right, although I do not mean to imply that they represent the ways in which menstruation is portrayed in sex education classes nationally.

11. Bahian lavatories are often equipped with a small, hand-held shower used to clean the body after excretion or during menstruation. Although I have not been able to find any information on the history of this object, it is clearly part of the modern hygienic arsenal for building an urban middle class.

12. Official recommendations state that IUDs can be inserted at any point in the cycle and do not limit this method to women who have already had children. Many of the doctors I met, however, continued to request that women come to the clinic during their menstrual periods for IUD insertions. Some explained that this was less painful for patients, or easier for them, whereas others claimed that women had been known to intentionally request an IUD insertion to provoke a miscarriage. This reveals the extent to which the IUD continues to be associated in multiple ways with abortion in Brazil, and the complex interplay between the uses patients make of biomedical practices and the shifting or informal protocols adopted that, in guiding and responding to these, shape popular ideas in a circular manner.

13. Leder's (1990, 92) project is to uncover a precultural basis to corporeal experience, or a "phenomenological invariant" that I have already suggested is deeply problematic. However, he simultaneously recognizes the importance of cultural factors in this process when he notes that "for the young and the aged, for adult women as opposed to men, normal body functioning includes regular and even extreme bodily shifts. Cultural prejudices lead us to forget or devalue such changes" (89).

Chapter 2: Is Menstruation Natural?

1. http://vivasemmenstruar.com.br (accessed June 11, 2013).

2. It is interesting to note that her scientific position is much more moderate and free of this type of language (e.g., Strassmann 1997).

3. "Uninterrupted use of hormonal contraceptives for menstrual suppression: why I do not recommend it," http://www.mum.org/soucas.htm (accessed June 11, 2014).

4. In Salvador, several doctors consented to give me interviews on the subject on the condition that their position would remain completely anonymous.

5. Two episodes gave PMS public visibility. In the early 1980s this diagnostic category was used as a mitigating circumstance for two British women in two separate murder trial cases. Both women received reduced sentences on the basis of a claim to diminished capacities due to PMS (see Law, Hey and Eagan 1985). The validity of PMS as a diagnostic category was publicly debated after "late luteal phase dysphoric disorder" (LLPDD) was included in the DSM-III in 1986. Following a letter-writing campaign by a coalition of feminist health professionals and the emergence of a debate between psychiatrists and gynecologists over which medical specialty was better suited to diagnose LLPDD, the diagnostic category was placed in an appendix under the heading "needing further study." Controversy reemerged in 1994 with the classification of premenstrual dysphoric disorder (PMDD) in the DSM-IV, opening the way to the use of fluoxetine hydrochloride (otherwise known as Prozac), under the name of Sarafem, for the treatment of "severe" cases of PMS (see Greenslit 2005).

6. For example, one woman I met used subdermal hormonal implants specifically to suppress menstruation—in view, she explained, of "controlling" her PMT—although she had had a tubal ligation and had no need for this method *as a contraceptive*. Of course many women do adopt menstrual-suppressive contraceptive methods specifically for their contraceptive function, and at times report putting up with the side effect of not bleeding because they appreciate the contraceptive efficacy of long-acting methods.

7. Cytotec is the commercial name for misoprostol, a prostaglandin used in the treatment of gastric ulcers. Because of the widespread use of Cytotec as an abortion-inducer in Brazil, a Ministry of Health resolution limited its commercialization to accredited hospitals. The drug is nevertheless still widely available on the black market. Guedes (2000) notes that an estimated 50 percent of the annual public health obstetrics budget was spent on treating botched abortions, but that the use of Cytotec (estimated in this study at 91 percent of all self-induced abortions, although the figure varies widely) has significantly reduced the number of postabortion complications, thereby decreasing overall maternal morbidity.

8. In *Regulating Menstruation* van de Walle and Renne (2001) outline how the definition and use of emmenagogues shift historically and contextually. However, regarding the menstrual regulating versus abortive use of emmenagogues, assumptions concerning women's "vague intentionality" run through the volume, at the expense of a more detailed ethnographic inquiry into how these are structured by legal and institutional

constraints. Santow (2001) provides elements of explanation in pointing to the fact that false consciousness and the publicized correcting of "irregularities and obstructions" were a "sinister" marketing strategy for abortifacients in early twentieth-century Euro-American contexts where abortion was criminalized.

9. In Brazil, medical councils, police, and health authorities all know about the private clinics, but nothing is done to close them because they serve the dominant, elite class, which tends to be above the law. In the current context of attempts to legalize abortion, religious and police authorities have had some of these closed, but they generally exist in remarkable impunity.

10. Here the semantic gap between "spontaneous" or "natural" on the one hand and "provoked" or "induced" on the other—that is, between nature and intervention—would be worthy of much greater analysis. In the testimonies I heard, women often reported strong emotion such as *susto* (fear) or shock or a fall, which were at times met by sardonic comments on behalf of medical staff (e.g., "I know the name of the demon that scared you: Cytotec!," as I once heard in a hospital).

11. Women often start with *chás*, because either they do not have the money to buy Cytotec or they drink these while they wait to obtain it. Chás used include alumã (*Vermonia baiensis*), espirradeira (*Nerium oleander*), and cravo (clove, *Syzgium aromaticum*). In a brief survey of substances available in the markets, I was also told of the efficacy of the "buchinha paulista" (*Luffa operculata*, a Cucurbitaceae) originary of Brazil. Various "recipes" were given, which involved boiling several times and distilling. The active properties of this plant are described as hemorrhagic and embryotoxic.

12. I was never told of this by women who recognized having used the methods themselves; it was always in reference to someone else's use, and tended to imply a degree of disapproval, conditioned by a strong local biomedical discourse concerning both the inappropriateness of provoking aborto and the danger of doing it in this manner.

13. In Judaism, physical contact between men and women is forbidden during menstruation and for one week after. At the end of this period, a woman takes a cleansing bath, called Mikvah, to mark the end of this ritually unclean period (Guterman 2006). Menstrual taboos within Christianity are one of the main reasons that have been used to keep women from positions of authority. In Islam, women's menstrual impurity is not considered contagious but menstruating women are not allowed to recite the Koran, enter a mosque, or pray or fast during Ramadan. Women are exempted from ritual obligations and festivities even if they desire to participate. Likewise, in Hinduism, women may not enter the puja room, cook, or occupy the same quarters as their kin during menstruation (Appfel-Marglin 1994). See also Montgomery (1974).

14. I am grateful to Haripriya Narasimhan for calling my attention to this.

15. Gillison (1993, 180–81) provides an exegesis of the elaborate rituals and prescriptions that Gimi follow to withhold menstrual blood, such as using ashes to seal the skin and make the body a perfect container of male fluids, transforming a woman from "*leaky bamboo*" to "*dusty taro*." The Gimi consider that menstrual blood is the blood of men. "A menstruating woman possesses something she *took from a man*" (180). Blood

songs are sung to arrest the menstrual flow. What is at stake is the fact that, for Gimi women, to withhold their menstrual blood is to express a desire to remain partheno-genetic. Gimi marital exchange rituals seek to displace the paternal presence inside a woman's body, replacing it with her husband's. Women live out this ambiguity, Gilli-son argues, because they recognize that the regeneration of life depends on these flows of male substance through their bodies. Berlin (1985) notes that the Aguaruna Jívaro of Perú use fertility regulators to achieve amenorrhea and reversible sterility, but she implies that they do so primarily because they hate menstruating, reporting that some Aguaruna women state that they become pregnant simply to avoid "the discomfort of menstruation" (139), a point that is not developed further. Weiner (1995, 166) notes that for the Foi of Papua New Guinea, impregnation (that is, the addition of semen to menstrual blood) is conceived of in terms of withholding or containing menstrual blood in the women's uterus, which makes it thick and *viscous* in contrast to the unre-strained *fluid* flow of menstrual blood, which has not been fastened by the accumula-tion of semen. The distinction between viscous and fluid is introduced to analyze Foi anxieties over uncontrollable flow of wealth. Indeed, the (Foi) parallel between the con-tinence of wealth and the continence of menstrual blood is marked by a distinction be-tween viscous (where wealth, energy, or substance is secured in the body of the clan/woman) and fluid (where it flows out). In Melanesia, a Strathernian reading would show blood has an origin in other persons, and withholding blood amounts to preventing the efficacy of others, blocking not just the blood (substance) but also its (social) source.

16. In a subsequent discussion she explained that she had been admitted to a hos-pital by emergency after she began to hemorrhage and was diagnosed with a fibroid "the size of a seven-month fetus." The doctors performed a full hysterectomy despite her young age. She explains this as the result of Oxum's (the Orixá who rules over the uterus) whim. After the hysterectomy, she recalls feeling an emptiness, "as a woman does after she gives birth," she added. Today she feels at peace with this, and jokes that she has enough *filhos emprestados* (borrowed children) to keep her busy.

17. Although I do not suggest that this is representative of the way the entire com-munity of Candomblé practitioners deals with menstruation, it was relayed by a signifi-cant number of persons.

Chapter 3: Sexing Hormones

1. I adopt here the Portuguese term and orthography because these correspond to the way travestis refer to themselves, in distinguishing themselves from transsexuals, transvestites, and gays. Part of the political claim of travestis is being recognized the right to be addressed as "she." Kulick's (1998) excellent ethnography gives a more de-tailed description of travesti sexual politics.

2. This was the way the president of ATRAS presented the situation to me.

3. At the time of writing I was not able to obtain information concerning the possi-bility for individuals to seek hormonal therapy without undergoing genital surgery for sex reassignment.

4. This is a reconstruction of her statement as it was made at the end of our meeting and was not recorded.

5. *Louca* (in the feminine, in Portuguese).

6. Transcript available from http://www.abc.net.au/catalyst/stories/s964127.htm (accessed September 14, 2015).

7. A term commonly used to evoke sexual desire.

8. This is not a transcribed statement since the questions were not recorded. These are practically, although not exactly, his words.

9. Some drugs have been so successful that the brand name has come to stand for their active principle, despite current ministry regulation that seeks to keep a check on the power of pharmaceutical laboratories by prohibiting the use of brand names in prescriptions, and thus making possible the prescription of generics or nationally produced "*similares*," which are nongeneric copies of patent drugs (see Sanabria 2014).

10. Schneider's *American Kinship* (1980 [1968]) revealed how blood signaled the shared biogenetic substance of relatedness, and as such evokes notions of fixity and permanence, which at times flowed through to the anthropological theories that grew out of this particular epistemology. The tension between the various meanings of blood, as a substance that can index both flow and fixity or immutability, has been analyzed by Carsten (2011). Likewise, Franklin (2001, 2013) examined the varied understandings that are carried by biological "facts" in the context of new biotechnological innovations that challenge the fixity of biological substance. Weston (1995) also noted the tension in meanings attributed to "biology" in Euro-American contexts, where the term is used to evoke immutability, despite the fact that it refers to the *changing* process of life.

11. She shows that, in male initiation, relations with women (mediated by milk) are substituted by relations with men (mediated by semen). By contrast, female initiation substitutes relations among women (mediated by milk) with relations with men, which in the context of marriage are mediated by semen (Strathern 1991, 203). But if, as she shows, semen cannot be considered quite as homogeneous as it is made to seem in Godelier's analysis, but takes male and female forms, then at best it can be said that the one, semen, encompasses the other, milk.

12. For a detailed description of the uses travestis make of industrial silicone, which is pumped directly into the body, see Kulick (1998).

13. This process involves the use of pharmaceutical sex hormones to induce multiple ovulations in women and then surgically retrieve the ova after monitoring their development, a highly invasive practice, unlike the collection of sperm.

Chapter 4: Hormonal Biopolitics

1. According to the 2006 PNDS census (analyzed in Perpétuo and Wong 2009), 75.7 percent of pills are obtained directly over the counter, often without prescription. A similar distribution was found for hormonal injections, with 74.9 percent of injections acquired directly in a pharmacy.

2. According to one of *Schering Brasil*'s regional sales representatives, Brazil is the

largest consumer of the hormonal IUD Mirena, with sales topping those in the United States.

3. Trimonthly injections such as Depo-Provera retail between US$5 and US$11. Mirena costs roughly US$200 plus medical honorariums (for a contraceptive efficacy of three to five years), and implants range widely in price from US$75–300 (for a contraceptive efficacy of six months to three years). See table I.1.

4. Two of three Brazilians lived in rural zones in 1950, against four of every five in urban centers by 1996 (Bozon 2005).

5. In 2006, 20.5 percent of women with at least eight years of schooling relied on sterilization, against 65.5 percent of women with no formal education (Perpétuo and Wong 2009, 93–94).

6. Depo-Provera has a troubling history worldwide. In the United States it was repeatedly denied Food and Drug Administration approval until 1992. Corea (personal communication) notes the lack of new evidence on the basis of which Depo-Provera was eventually approved and points to the way it is targeted to minority or institutionalized women (Corea 1980). See also Kaler (1998) for an analysis of Depo-Provera's 1981 ban in Zimbabwe.

7. *Secretaria Estadual de Saúde da Bahia* (SESAB).

8. This estimation was achieved by counting the number of units distributed in each health post over one month (October 2008). The disparity between this figure and figures on injection use for the population as a whole can be explained according to a range of factors. First, the PNDS 2006 data (discussed in Perpétuo and Wong 2009) take into account all women, as opposed to women using some form of contraception, as is the case when sampling in a family planning unit. Second, this estimation is made in an urban setting (the authors of the report accompanying the PNDS 2006 study note that this study oversampled in rural areas). Third, arrivals vary from one month to the other. Finally, it reveals that hormonal injections are disproportionally represented in public health units.

9. Brazil is a federal state comprising twenty-seven regional states, including Bahia. The National Ministry of Health in Brasília devolves resources and oversees the actions of the regional state health secretaries.

10. During my fieldwork, family planning ambulatórios in public maternity units were being discontinued because the activity was being transferred to the newly established neighborhood basic health units (BHUs). The availability of services in BHUs varied widely (some were functional, whereas others consisted of nothing more than four walls), and, at the very best, gynecological and family planning consultations were limited to one day a week, and methods were completely lacking in many. Although the problem was explained as a temporary one, it had been going on for roughly two years when I arrived and continued throughout my fieldwork.

11. The collection of statistics on health has a long history in Brazil, beginning with the General Direction of Statistics (1871) and the creation of the National Department of Statistics (1934), which became the Brazilian Institute of Geography and Statistics two years later (http://www.ibge.gov.br/home/disseminacao/eventos/missao

/instituicao.shtm, accessed July 14, 2013). IBGE is a national entity, whereas DATASUS is part of the Ministry of Health. DATASUS presents its mission as founded on the collection and treatment of information through which the coordination of health services can be administered. Here, data management is pitched as integral to the "democratization of health" through facilitating the decentralization of services and the management of resources (www.datasus.gov.br, my translation).

12. The specific objectives of the *Programa de Humanização do Pré-Natal e Nascimento* are to recruit pregnant women, guarantee their access to different health services, establish a link between prenatal care and delivery, and guarantee quality of assistance in both the prenatal period (realization of clinical exams: antigens [ABO, Rh], urine, glycemia, hemoglobin/hematocrit, HIV) and assistance to the newborn (including immunization).

13. Goldstein (2003) deals with the question of humor in Brazil in her ethnography *Laughter Out of Place*, and Scheper-Hughes (1992) touches on the question in her discussion of violence in everyday life.

14. Given the extremely high rate of female sterilization in Brazil, many services place restrictions (age and number of children) on who can obtain a tubal ligation. Interestingly, although I do not have sufficient space to develop this here, a significant proportion of the "myths" that medical professionals work to dispel find their origin in medical practice. Many of the things that women expected in the encounters were based on old medical protocols that had evolved but remained in the public imaginary, as it were. As medical norms shift, what is taken as ignorance is often simply expertise in older ways of doing things.

15. Women in Brazil tend to count all their pregnancies as children they have had, and specify how many are living. This includes children who were born but died and pregnancies that were interrupted in deliberate or accidental ways.

16. Following accusations of excessive female sterilizations, the ambulatórios I visited established limits on who could access this procedure, such that each day, several women would present themselves requesting sterilization and be turned down on the basis of their young age.

17. Although my experience of selecting vasectomy candidates is limited to CEPARH.

18. I make a rapid retrospective calculation: both women became pregnant in February, the Carnival of his twenty-first year.

19. This, however, may be a bias produced by my presence, or by the fact that CEPARH has been the target of accusations concerning their overly enthusiastic interventions in family planning among low-income segments of the population. During the period of my fieldwork, CEPARH female sterilizations were performed only one day a week.

20. The fact that hormonal implants are, in Brazil, limited to the private sector is reflected in the low distribution of this method for the population as a whole. Implant use accounted for only 0.1 percent of all women. Users of hormonal implants were all found to have nine years of study or more (Perpétuo and Wong 2009, 136), which confirms that this method is predominantly adopted by middle- and upper-class women.

21. Despite what Bahian doctors often tell their patients, there is little or no epidemiological evidence establishing links between observed behavior changes (such as increased sexual activity), or even differences in subjective mood assessments (such as increased sexual pleasure), and the use of synthetic sex steroids.

22. Likewise, in Brazil, sexual mores were of great concern to hygienist reformers of the early twentieth century. While gratuitous sexual pleasure was reprimanded, according to medical historian J. F. Costa (2004, 222), sex was medicalized within marital relations "not for its excesses, but for its deficiencies." This phrase, taken from a medical thesis defended in Rio de Janeiro in 1842, reveals that these questions are anything but new.

23. In the United Kingdom, Schering's "Women feel well on Yasmin" marketing strategy was deemed misleading on eleven separate counts in a Prescription Medicines Code of Practice Authority (PMCPA) ruling on November 22, 2002. The ruling concluded that there is no compelling published evidence to suggest that Yasmin offers any advantages over other, longer-established combined oral contraceptives with regard to weight gain, skin condition, or premenstrual symptoms. It argued that the claim that Yasmin "is the pill for well-being" is unjustified and misleading and should be withdrawn, and pointed to the fact that Yasmin's effects on venous thromboembolic disease had not been quantified (Drug and Therapeutics Bulletin exposes Medicines Control Agency Incompetence, Press Release by Consumers' Association UK, December 8, 2002).

24. In their study, Menezes et al. (2006) clearly relate pregnancy outcomes to inequalities in health care provision among different social categories within Brazil (class and regional). They found that although early pregnancy was rarer among the socially privileged groups they studied, the rate of abortion was higher, indicating that when pregnancy did occur, abortion was the most likely outcome. For low-income women with less schooling, they show, pregnancy is more frequent, and becoming a mother is considered a viable life project.

25. The degradation of the active principle by the liver, requiring the administration of higher doses when administered orally.

26. Before the establishment of the SUS in 1988, formal employment gave access to medical services through the National Institute of Medical Assistance and Social Providence, a system that excluded those in the informal sector of the economy.

27. I am grateful to Ashley Lebner for the stimulating conversations that helped me develop this point.

Chapter 5: Sex Hormones

1. In his ethnography of pharmaceutical sales practices, salesperson-turned-anthropologist Oldani (2004) remarks on the importance of strategic gifting in pharmaceutical marketing. This gift economy, into which pharmaceutical corporations invest billions of dollars, serves to craft relations with doctors and gauge promotional strategies as well as generate sales.

2. The strategic potential of off-label uses was in fact already evident to the early pill developers, such as Katherine MacCormick, who understood that the 1957 FDA approval of Enovid for gynecological disorders would certainly lead women to use it as a contraceptive (Tone 2001). Indeed, in 1960 the FDA approved Enovid as a contraceptive.

3. A particularly telling example of how the arbitrages made by insurance companies inscribe specific gendered politics into pharmaceuticals is given by Tone (2001, 291), who notes that the US$10-per-pill Viagra was willingly covered by American insurance companies, while the much cheaper oral contraceptive pill is not.

4. http://www.elmeco.com.br/categoria/produtos/, accessed May 16, 2014.

5. A fact that they attributed to their own carelessness and were highly reluctant to discuss further. They simply noted that as part of the quality control of the lab, they have regular blood hormone concentration tests, and these are "outside the norm." But they laughed the problem away, joking that one was sterilized and the other had undergone menopause, so what did it matter anyway?

6. In a study reported by Coutinho and Montgomery (1999), loss of libido is a common side effect, which is why, at CEPARH, elcometrine and testosterone are commonly associated.

7. His own vision of "Women's Hormonal Intelligence: How the Menstrual Cycle Can Be an Ally and Not an Enemy of the Feminine Balance" (Berenstein 2001) equally naturalizes social roles and characteristics attributed to hormones.

8. Although to state this is to accept in a problematically straightforward manner the idea that hormonal categories (estrogens, androgens, and so on) have specific effects on sexual desire, a question that is very much open, despite my recognition of the tangibility and "materiality" of hormonal effects.

9. "Implantes Hormonias," http://www.elsimarcoutinho.com/implantes-hormonais /beneficios-a-mulher/?lang=pt (accessed May 16, 2014; my translation).

10. "A Mágica dos hormônios: hormônios da felicidade," *Marie Claire*, no. 169, April 2005.

11. http://boaforma.abril.com.br/famosas/famosas-em-boa-forma/carla-regina-em agreceu-5-kg-532732.shtml, December 2012, accessed October 17, 2013.

12. No. 484: February 2013 (http://revistaplaneta.terra.com.br/edicao/484).

13. As a contrast one could point to the recent sanitary crisis in France around third- and fourth-generation pills, itself occurring much later than the British one.

14. See Peterson (2014) for an eloquent discussion of how the existence of regulation in North America and Western Europe is dependent on its absence elsewhere.

15. For a critique of such an approach see Henare, Holbraad, and Wastell (2007).

16. According to Bayer, drospirenone is still under patent. In 2005 the Brazilian pharmaceutical laboratory Libbs registered Elaní with ANVISA and immediately faced a trial by Schering for patent infringement. Libbs retaliated on several fronts: It claimed that Schering's drospirenone patent no. 1101055–0 relies on technology described in patent DE 3.022.337, registered in 1980 and therefore in the public domain. Further, given the fact that Elaní is packaged as an extended-regime pill, Libbs claimed to have innovated on and not just "copied" Yasmin. After two Brazilian rulings denied Libbs's

request to suspend Schering's patent, Libbs took the issue to the Brazilian Supreme Tribunal of Justice, and to this day, Schering's patent has not been annulled, nor has Libbs been formally allowed or legally impeded from commercializing Elaní. See Sanabria (2014) for more details.

17. This fact is by no means unanimous. Some women, particularly those troubled by swelling and weight gain, made a clear relation between the hormonal composition of oral and nonoral steroid contraceptives.

18. The degradation of the active principle by the liver, requiring the administration of higher doses when administered orally.

Conclusion: Limits That Do Not Foreclose

1. Nick Shapiro's *At Home in the Surreal* inspired this formulation (paper presented at the Embodied Being, Environing World: Local Biologies and Local Ecologies in Global Health workshop in Paris, June 5–6, 2014).

2. Likewise, in the epilogue to *Organism and the Origin of Self*, Dorion Sagan and Lynn Margulis (1991) examine how scientific reductionism coupled with the "pervasive influence of IndoEuropean grammar," with its subject–verb–object structures, works to produce an image of the topologically enclosed body as the locus for "self." Resisting such a view, which is grounded in an idea of the organism that is ontological rather than biological, they argue that bodies are malleable and that the membranes that enclose them are better thought of as "constantly changing semi-permeable barriers" rather than as "a concrete, literal, self-possessed wall."

3. The problem I am attempting to underscore here pertains less to van de Port's analysis, which I am deeply sympathetic with, and more to the history of our discipline.

4. Though the economic and societal events that have marked Western Europe and North America over the past decade have concomitantly produced a vision of this version of modernity as having reached its apex and tipped over into a form of decadence.

5. This is further compounded by the fact that I finalize this text in (American) English from France, where I am now institutionally based. Having been trained in the United Kingdom, the implicit term in my comparative endeavor thus shifts — at times a little crudely — between the different nationally shared assumptions and academic conventions of these places.

6. This, of course, is not a new insight, as we know from what Boesoou, a man in New Caledonia, told Leenhardt in the early twentieth century: what missionarization brought was not the idea of the soul but that of the body (see Breton et al. 2006).

7. Castro-Klarén (2000) sees this as an inherent contradiction of *Antropófagia*, which as a move implies a domestication of the latent violence of the asymmetrical relations — both internal and external — that Brazilian elites sustain.

8. As far as I am aware, the preface to the new edition is not translated into English.

9. Which, interestingly, in French is a term that does not distinguish sensing matter from meaning, so there may be issues of translation at stake in this debate.

10. To quote the passage in full:

The parallax Real is thus opposed to the standard (Lacanian) notion of the Real as that which "always returns to its place"—as that which remains the same in all possible (symbolic) universes: the parallax Real is, rather, that which accounts for the very *multiplicity* of appearances of the same underlying Real—it is not the hard core which persists as the Same, but the hard bone of contention which pulverizes the sameness into the multitude of appearances. In a first move, the Real is the impossible hard core which we cannot confront directly, but only through the lenses of a multitude of symbolic fictions, virtual formations. In a second move, this very hard core is purely virtual, actually non-existent, an X which can be reconstructed only retroactively, from the multitude of symbolic formations which are "all that there actually is." (Žižek 2006, 26)

11. Another critique of Malabou's neurobiological interpretation that I have not encountered might have focused on the remarkable primacy she continues to give to the brain and the central nervous system—as opposed to the mindful body—and to the distinctions between mind and body that this brain-centered focus unwittingly reproduces. There is much scope to extend her analysis of neuroplasticity well beyond the neural brain, to what Pert (2003) called the "chemical brain," for example.

12. It would be interesting to explore this in relation to Taussig's observation that in the context of Colombia's violent *narco* wars, horrific stories circulate concerning the failures of what he calls cosmic surgeries (or "soul lifts"). Can this fascinating moment he describes be understood as the counterbalancing of a previous fascination with the penultimateness and continual nonending of changeabilities? A collective public interest in the explosive cost of plastic surgeries in the era of Bataillian *dépense*?

REFERENCES

Abrahamsson, Sebastian, and Bertoni Filippo. 2014. "Compost Politics: Experimenting with Togetherness in Vermicomposting." *Environmental Humanities* 4: 125–48.

Adams, Vincanne, and Stacy Pigg, eds. 2005. *Sex in Development: Science, Sexuality and Morality in Global Perspective*. Durham, NC: Duke University Press.

Akrich, Madeleine. 1996. Le Médicament comme objet technique. *Revue internationale de Psychopathologie* 21: 135–58.

Alves, Maria Teresa Seabra Soares de Britto e, T. V. Barreto de Araújo, Thália V. Barreto de Alves, Sandra Valongueiro Alves, Lillian F. B. Marinho, Eleonora Schiavo, Greice Menezes, Liberata Campos Coimbra, Cláudia Teresa Frias Rios, Ana Cláudia Rodrigues, Ulla Macedo Romeu, Estela M. L. Aquino, Luci Praciano Lim. 2014. "Atenção ao aborto no Sistema Único de Saúde no Nordeste Brasileiro: a estrutura dos serviços." *Revista Brasileira de Saúde Materno Infantil* 14 (3): 229–39.

Amaral, Maria Clara Estanislau do. 2003. "Percepção e significado da menstruação para as mulheres." MA diss., Faculty of Medical Sciences, Universidade Estadual de Campinas.

Apffel-Marglin, F. 1994. "The Sacred Groves." *Manushi* (82): 22–32.

Appadurai, Arjun. 2006. "The Thing Itself." *Public Culture* 18 (1): 15–21.

Appadurai, Arjun, ed. 1986. *The Social Life of Things: Commodities in Cultural Perspective*. New York: Cambridge University Press.

Aquino, Estela. 2014. "Reinventing Delivery and Childbirth in Brazil: Back to the Future." *Cadernos de Saúde Pública* 30 (1): S8–10.

Aquino, Estela, Maria Luiza Heilborn, Daniela Knauth, Michel Bozon, Maria da Conceição, Jenny Araújo, and Greice Menezes. 2003. "Adolescência e reprodução no Brasil: a heterogeneidade dos perfis sociais." *Cadernos de Saúde Pública* 19 (Suppl. 2): S377–88.

Aquino, Estela, Greice M. S. Menezes, Thália V. Barreto-de-Araújo, Maria Teresa Alves, Maria da Conceição C. Almeida, Sandra Valongueiro Alves, Francisca Eleonora Schiavo, Lilian F. B. Marinho, Liberata C. Coimbra, and Michael E. Reichenheim. 2014. "Quality Assessment of Treatment Associated with Abortion: A Prototype Questionnaire for Health Services Users." *Cadernos de Saúde Pública* 30 (9): 2005–16.

Aquino, Estela M. L., Greice Menezes, Thália Velho Barreto-de-Araújo, Maria Teresa Alves, Sandra Valongueiro Alves, Maria da Conceição Chagas de Almeida, Eleonora Schiavo, Luci Praciano Lima, Carlos Augusto Santos de Menezes, Lilian Fátima Barbosa Marinho, Liberata Campos Coimbra, and Oona Campbell. 2012. "Qualidade da atenção ao aborto no Sistema Único de Saúde do Nordeste brasileiro: o que dizem as mulheres?" *Ciência & Saúde Coletiva* 17 (7): 1765–76.

Association of Reproductive Health Professionals. 2006. "Survey Reveals Confusion about Menstruation." Press release. Accessed September 15, 2015. http://www.arhp .org/modules/press/SURVEY-REVEALS-CONFUSION-ABOUT-MENSTRUATION -ABOUNDS—/15.

Association of Reproductive Health Professionals. 2004a. "Extended and Continuous Use of Contraceptives to Reduce Menstruation." *Clinical Proceedings of the Association of Reproductive Health Professionals.* September 2004.

Association of Reproductive Health Professionals. 2004b. "Taking Charge of Menstruation: New Options for Women." *Health and Sexuality* 9 (1).

Bahamondes, Luis, and M. Valeria Bahamondes. 2014. "New and Emerging Contraceptives: A State-of-the-Art Review." *International Journal of Women's Health* 6: 221–34.

Baillargeon, J. P., D. K. McClish, P. A. Essah, and J. E. Nestler. 2005. "Association between the Current Use of Low-Dose Oral Contraceptives and Cardiovascular Arterial Disease: A Meta-analysis." *Journal of Clinical Endocrinology and Metabolism* 90 (7): 3863–70.

Bakhtin, Mikhail. 1984. *Rabelais and His World*, translated by Hélène Iswolsky. Bloomington: Indiana University Press.

Bancroft, John. 1995. "The Menstrual Cycle and the Well Being of Women." *Social Science and Medicine* 41 (6): 785–91.

Barad, Karen. 2007. *Meeting the Universe Halfway: Quantum Physics and the Entanglement of Matter and Meaning.* Durham, NC: Duke University Press.

Barbosa, R. M., E. M. Aquino, M. L. Heilborn, and E. Berquó, eds. 2002. *Interfaces: Gênero, Sexualidade e Saúde Reproductiva.* São Paolo: Editora UNICAMP.

Barry, Andrew. 2005. "Pharmaceutical Matters: The Invention of Informed Materials." *Theory, Culture and Society* 22 (1): 51–69.

Belaunde, Luisa Elvira. 2005. *El recuerdo de Luna: Género, sangre y memoria entre los pueblos amazónicos.* Lima: Fondo Editorial do Banco Central de Reserva del Perú.

Beltrán, Carlos López. 2007. "Hippocratic Bodies. Temperament and Castas in Spanish America (1570–1820)." *Journal of Spanish Cultural Studies* 8 (2): 253–89.

BEMFAM, IBGE, Ministério da Saúde, DHS, USAID, FNUAP, and UNICEF. 1996. *Pesquisa Nacional Sobre Demografia e Saúde*. Rio de Janeiro: Publicação BEMFAM/DHS.

Berenstein, Elizer. 2001. *A Inteligência Hormonal da Mulher*. Rio de Janeiro: Editora Objetiva Ltda.

Berlin, Elois Ann. 1985. "Aspects of Fertility Regulation among the Aguaruna Jívaro of Perú." In *Women's Medicine: Cross-Cultural Studies of Indigenous Fertility Regulation*, edited by Newman Lucile, 125–46. New Brunswick, NJ: Rutgers University Press.

Biehl, João. 2005. *Vita: Life in a Zone of Social Abandonment*. Berkeley: University of California Press.

Biehl, João. 2004. "The Activist State: Global Pharmaceuticals, AIDS, and Citizenship in Brazil." *Social Text* 22 (3): 105–32.

Biehl, João, and Adriana Petryna. 2013. "Legal Remedies: Therapeutic Markets and the Judicialization of the Right to Health." In *When People Come First: Critical Studies in Global Health*, edited by João Biehl and Adriana Petryna, 325–46. Princeton, NJ: Princeton University Press.

Bilenky, Thais. 2012. "O 'Chip' da Beleza. Equilíbrio." *Folha de S. Paulo*, November 27, 2012.

Boltanski, Luc, and Eve Chiapello. 1999. *Le nouvel esprit du capitalisme*. Paris: Gallimard (Nrf Essais).

Bonneuil, Christophe, and Jean-Baptiste Fressoz. 2013. *L'Evénement Anthropocène: La Terre, l'histoire et nous*. Paris: Seuil.

Bozon, Michel. 2005. "L'évolution des scénarios de la vie reproductive des femmes au Brésil. Médicalisation, genre et ingalités sociales." *Tiers-Monde* 46 (182): 359–84.

Breton, Stéphane, Michèle Coquet, Michael Houseman, Jean-Marie Schaeffer, Anne-Christine Taylor, and Eduardo Viveiros de Castro. 2006. *Qu'est Ce Qu'un Corps?* Paris: Flammarion, Musée du Quai Branly.

Browner, Carole. 1985. "Traditional Techniques for Diagnosis, Treatment and Control of Pregnancy in Cali, Colombia." In *Women's Medicine: Cross-Cultural Studies of Indigenous Fertility Regulation*, edited by Lucile F. Newman and James M. Nyce, 99–123. New Brunswick, NJ: Rutgers University Press.

Browner, Carole, and Carolyn Sargent, eds. 2011. *Reproduction, Globalization and the State: New Theoretical and Ethnographic Perspectives*. Durham, NC: Duke University Press.

Brumberg, Joan. 1993. "'Something Happens to Girls': Menarche and the Emergence of the Modern American Hygienic Imperative." *Journal of the History of Sexuality* 4 (1): 99–127.

Brynhildsen, Jan. 2014. "Combined Hormonal Contraceptives: Prescribing Patterns, Compliance, and Benefits versus Risks." *Therapeutic Advances in Drug Safety* 5 (5): 201–13.

Buchwald, Henry, and Danette Oien. 2013. "Metabolic/Bariatric Surgery Worldwide 2011." *Obesity Surgery* 23 (4): 427–36.

Buckley, Thomas, and Alma Gottlieb, eds. 1988. *Blood Magic: The Anthropology of Menstruation*. Berkeley: University of California Press.

Butler, Judith. 1993. *Bodies That Matter: On the Discursive Limits of "Sex."* New York: Routledge.

Butler, Judith. 1988. *Gender Trouble: Feminism and the Subversion of Identity.* New York: Routledge.

Butler, Judith, and Catherine Malabou. 2010. *Sois mon corps: Une lecture contemporaine de la domination et de la servitude chez Hegel.* Paris: Éditions Bayard.

Bynum, Caroline Walker. 1991. *Fragmentation and Redemption: Essays on Gender and the Human Body in Medieval Religion.* New York: Urzone Publishers.

Caldeira, Teresa. 2000. *City of Walls: Crime, Segregation and Citizenship in São Paulo.* Berkeley: University of California Press.

Carsten, Janet. 2011. "Substance and Relationality: Blood in Contexts." *Annual Review of Anthropology* 40: 19–35.

Castro-Klarén, Sara. 2000. "A Genealogy for the 'Manifesto Antropofago,' or the Struggle between Socrates and the Caraibe." *Nepantla: Views from South* 1 (2): 295–322.

Cibula, D., A. Gompel, A. O. Mueck, C. La Vecchia, P. C. Hannaford, S. O. Skouby, M. Zikan, and L. Dusek. 2010. "Hormonal Contraception and Risk of Cancer." *Human Reproduction Update* 16 (6): 631–50.

Clarke, Adele, Laura Mamo, Jennifer Fosket, and Janet Shim, eds. 2010. *Biomedicalization: Technoscience, Health, and Illness in the U.S.* Durham, NC: Duke University Press.

Clifton, Donna, Toshiko Kaneda, and Lori Ashford. 2008. Family Planning Worldwide 2008 Data Sheet. Population Reference Bureau. Accessed February 6, 2015. http://www.prb.org/Publications/Datasheets/2008/familyplanningworldwide.aspx.

Cohen, Lawrence. 2005. "Operability, Bioavailability, and Exception." In *Global Assemblages: Technology, Politics and Ethics as Anthropological Problems*, edited by Aihwa Ong and Stephen Collier, 79–90. Oxford: Blackwell.

Corea, Gena. 1980. "The Depo-Provera Weapon." In *Birth Control and Controlling Birth: Women-Centred Perspectives*, edited by Helen Holmes, Betty Hoskins, and Michael Gross, 107–16. Totowa, NJ: Humana Press.

Corrêa, Marilena. 2001. *Novas Technologias Reprodutivas: Limites da biologia ou biologia sem limites?* Rio de Janeiro: Editora da UERJ.

Corrêa, Sonia. 1998. "Anticoncepcionais injetáveis na perspectiva feminista: O debate histórico e os novos desafios." In *Políticas, Mercado, Ética: Demandas e desafios no campo da saúde reprodutiva*, edited by Margareth Arilha and Maria Teresa Citeli, 25–42. São Paulo: Editora 34 Ltda.

Costa, Ana Maria. 2009. "Participação social na conquista das políticas de saúde para mulheres no Brasil." *Ciência & Saúde Coletiva* 14 (4): 1073–83.

Costa, Jurandir Freire. [1979] 2004. *Ordem Médica e Norma Familiar*, 5th ed. Rio de Janeiro: Edições Graal Ltda.

Coutinho, Elsimar. 2007. "To Bleed or Not Bleed, That Is the Question." *Contraception* 76: 263–66.

Coutinho, Elsimar. 2004. *Informe Técnico: Implantes.* Salvador: CEPARH.

Coutinho, Elsimar, and Malcolm Montgomery. 1999. "Elcometrine for Long-Term

Contraception and Clinical Management of Endometriosis." In *Reproductive Medicine: A Millennium Review. Proceedings of the 10th World Congress of Human Reproduction*, edited by E. Coutinho and P. Spinola. New York: Parthenon Publishing Group.

Coutinho, Elsimar, with Sheldon Segal. 1999. *Is Menstruation Obsolete? How Suppressing Menstruation Can Help Women Who Suffer from Anemia, Endometriosis, or PMS*. Oxford: Oxford University Press.

Crabbé, P., E. Diczfalusy, and C. Djerassi. 1980. "Injectable Contraceptive Synthesis: An Example of International Cooperation." *Science* 209: 992–94.

Cruz, Elaine. 2014. "Preço da cesta básica cai em 11 capitais, diz Dieese." EBC Agência Brasil. Accessed July 20, 2015. http://agenciabrasil.ebc.com.br/economia/noticia /2014-10/preco-da-cesta-basica-cai-em-11-capitais-diz-dieese.

DaMatta, Roberto. 1991. *Carnivals, Rogues, and Heroes: An Interpretation of the Brazilian Dilemma*, translated by John Drury. Notre Dame, IN: University of Notre Dame Press.

DaMatta, Roberto. 1987. *A Casa e a Rua: Espaço, cidadania, mulher e morte no Brasil*. Rio de Janeiro: Editora Guanabara.

Daniels, Kimberly, William Mosher, and Jo Jones. 2013. "Contraceptive Methods Women Have Ever Used: United States, 1982–2010." National Health Statistics Reports. Centers for Disease Control and Prevention. Number 62, February 14.

Da Silva, Ligia, Luis de Souza, J. P. Cerdeira, Cristiane Pinto, and Renata Oliveira. 1997. "Algumas características do setor privado de saúde de Salvador, Bahia, Brasil." *Cadernos de Saúde Pública* 13 (4): 701–9.

de Bastos, M., B. H. Stegeman, F. R. Rosendaal, A. Van Hylckama Vlieg, F. M. Helmerhorst, T. Stijnen, O. M. Dekkers. 2014. "Combined Oral Contraceptives: Venous Thrombosis." *Cochrane Database of Systematic Reviews* (3): CD010813. doi: 10.1002/ 14651858.CD010813.pub2.

DeGrandpre, Richard. 2006. *The Cult of Pharmacology: How America Became the World's Most Troubled Drug Culture*. Durham, NC: Duke University Press.

De la Bellacasa, Maria Puig. 2011. "Matters of Care in Technoscience: Assembling Neglected Things." *Social Studies of Science* 41: 85–106. doi: 10.1177/0306312710380301.

de Laet, Marianne, and Annemarie Mol. 2000. "The Zimbabwe Bush Pump: Mechanics of a Fluid Technology." *Social Studies of Science* 30 (2): 225–63.

DeLoughery, Thomas. 2011. "Estrogen and Thrombosis: Controversies and Common Sense. *Reviews in Endocrine and Metabolic Disorders* (12): 77–84.

den Tonkelaar, I., and B. J. Oddens. 1999. "Preferred Frequency and Characteristics of Menstrual Bleeding in Relation to Reproductive Status, Oral Contraceptive Use, and Hormone Replacement Therapy Use." *Contraception* 59: 357–62.

De Zordo, Silvia. 2012. "Programming the Body, Planning Reproduction, Governing Life: The '(Ir-)rationality' of Family Planning and the Embodiment of Social Inequalities in Salvador da Bahia (Brazil)." *Anthropology and Medicine* 19 (2): 207–23.

Diniz, Simone. 2012. "Materno-Infantilism, Feminism and Maternal Health Policy in Brazil." *Reproductive Health Matters* 20 (39): 125–32.

Dos Reis, Ana Paula. 2002. *A concepção hormonal do corpo: Fisiologia e comportamento feminino na menopausa*. 26th Annual Meeting of ANPOCS, October 22–26, 2002, Caxambu.

Douglas, Mary. [1966] 2002. *Purity and Danger: An Analysis of Concepts of Pollution and Taboo*. London: Routledge Classics.

Douglas, Mary. [1975] 1999. *Implicit Meanings: Selected Essays in Anthropology*. 2nd ed. New York: Routledge.

Douglas, Mary. 1970. *Natural Symbols: Explorations in Cosmology*. London: Barrie and Rockliff.

Duarte, Luis Fernando Dias. 1999. "A medicina e o médico na boca do povo." *Revista Antropológicas* 9: 7–14.

Duarte, Luis Fernando Dias. 1986. *Da vida nervosa nas classes trabalhadoras urbanas*. Rio de Janeiro: Zahar.

Duden, Barbara. 1991. *The Woman beneath the Skin: A Doctor's Patients in Eighteenth-Century Germany*. Cambridge, MA: Harvard University Press.

Dumit, Joseph. 2012. *Drugs for Life: How Pharmaceutical Companies Define Our Health*. Durham, NC: Duke University Press.

Ecks, Stefan. 2005. "Pharmaceutical Citizenship: Antidepressant Marketing and the Promise of Demarginalization in India." *Anthropology and Medicine* 12 (3): 239–54.

Edelman, A., E. Micks, M. F. Gallo, J. T. Jensen, and D. A. Grimes. 2014. "Continuous or Extended Cycle vs. Cyclic Use of Combined Hormonal Contraceptives for Contraception." *Cochrane Database of Systematic Reviews* (7): CD004695. doi: 10.1002/14651858.CD004695.pub3.

Edelman, Alison, Robyn Lewa, Carrie Cwiakb, Mark Nicholsa, and Jeffrey Jensena. 2007. "Acceptability of Contraceptive-Induced Amenorrhea in a Racially Diverse Group of US Women." *Contraception* 75 (6): 450–53.

Edmonds, Alex. 2013. "The Biological Subject of Aesthetic Medicine." *Feminist Theory* 14 (1): 65–82.

Edmonds, Alex. 2010. *Pretty Modern: Beauty, Sex and Plastic Surgery in Brazil*. Durham, NC: Duke University Press.

Edmonds, Alex. 2007. "'The Poor Have the Right to Be Beautiful': Cosmetic Surgery in Neoliberal Brazil." *Journal of the Royal Anthropological Institute* 13 (2): 363–81.

Edmonds, Alex, and Emilia Sanabria. 2014. "Medical Borderlands: Engineering the Body with Plastic Surgery and Hormonal Therapies in Brazil." *Anthropology and Medicine*. Special issue: "Mediating Medical Technologies: Flows and Frictions of New Socialities." 21 (2): 202–16.

Elias, Norbert. 1994. *The Civilizing Process*, translated by Edmund Jephcott. Oxford: Blackwell.

EngenderHealth. 2002. *Contraceptive Sterilization: Global Issues and Trends*. New York: EngenderHealth Publications. Accessed on September 15, 2015. https://www.engenderhealth.org/pubs/family-planning/contraceptive-sterilization-factbook.php.

Estanislau do Amaral, M. C., E. Hardy, E. M. Hebling, and A. Faúndes. 2005. "Menstruation and Amenorrhea: Opinion of Brazilian Women." *Contraception* 72: 157–61.

Etkin, Nina. 1992. "'Side Effects': Cultural Constructions and Reinterpretations of Western Pharmaceuticals." *Medical Anthropology Quarterly* 6 (2): 99–113.

Faircloth, C. 2013. *Militant Lactivism?: Attachment Parenting and Intensive Motherhood in the UK and France*. Oxford: Berghahn Books.

Faria, Nula, and Maria Silveira, eds. 2000. *Mulheres, Corpo e Saude*. São Paolo: Semprevía Organização Feminista (SOF).

Fausto-Sterling, Anne. 2000. *Sexing the Body: Gender Politics and the Construction of Sexuality*. New York: Basic Books.

Faveret Filho, P., and P. Oliveira. 1989. *A universalização excludente: Reflexões sobre a tendência do sistema de saúde*. Rio de Janeiro: UERJ/IEI.

Ferreroa, Simone, Luiza Helena Abbamontea, Margherita Giordanoa, Franco Alessandria, Paola Anserinia, Valentino Remorgidaa, and Nicola Ragnia. 2006. "What Is the Desired Menstrual Frequency of Women without Menstruation-Related Symptoms?" *Contraception* 73: 537–41.

Figoli, Moema. 2006. "Evolução da educação no Brasil: Uma análise das taxas entre 1970 e 2000 segundo o grau da última série concluída." *Revista Brasileira de Estudos de População* 23 (1): 129–50.

Fitzgerald, Des, and Felicity Callard. 2015. "Social Science and Neuroscience Beyond Interdisciplinarity: Experimental Entanglements." *Theory, Culture and Society* 32 (1): 3–32.

Fort, Catherine. 2001. "Financing Contraceptive Supplies in Developing Countries: Summary of Issues, Options, and Experience." Series: Meeting the Challenge: Securing Contraceptive Supplies. A joint publication of John Snow Inc. (JSI), Population Action International (PAI), the Program for Appropriate Technology in Health (PATH) and Wallace Global Fund, Washington, DC, edited by C. Hart, R. Moore, and P. Dougherty. http://www.populationaction.org/Publications/Reports /Meeting_the_Challenge/ asset_upload_file856_5487.pdf (accessed July 11, 2010).

Fortun, Kim. 2012. "Ethnography in Late Industrialism." *Cultural Anthropology* 27 (3): 446–64.

Foucault, Michel. [1963] 2003. *Naissance de la clinique*. Paris: PUF.

Foucault, Michel. 1976. *Histoire de la sexualité I: La volonté de savoir*. Paris: Gallimard.

Frank, Robert. 1931. "The Hormonal Causes of Premenstrual Tension." *Archives of Neurology and Psychiatry* 26 (5): 1053–57.

Franklin, Sarah. 2014. "Analogic Return: The Reproductive Life of Conceptuality." *Theory, Culture and Society* 31 (2–3): 243–61.

Franklin, Sarah. 2013. *Biological Relatives: IVF, Stem Cells and the Future of Kinship*. Durham, NC: Duke University Press.

Franklin, Sarah, and Margaret Lock, eds. 2003. *Remaking Life and Death: Toward an Anthropology of the Biosciences*. Santa Fe, NM: School of American Research Press.

Franklin, Sarah, and Helena Ragone, eds. 1998. *Reproducing Reproduction: Kinship, Power, and Technological Innovation*. Philadelphia: University of Pennsylvania Press.

Freyre, Gilberto. [1933] 1990. *Casa-grande e senzala : Formação da família brasileira sob o regime de economia patriarcal*. Lisboa: Coleção Livros do Brasil.

Fry, Peter. 2000. "Politics, Nationality, and the Meanings of 'Race' in Brazil." *Daedalus* 129 (2): 83–118.

Galvão, L., and J. Diaz. eds. 1999. *Saúde Sexual e Reproductiva no Brasil: Dilemas e Desafios*. São Paolo: Hucitec, Population Council.

Gaudillière, J. P. 2004. "Hormones, régimes d'innovation et stratégies d'entreprise: Les exemples de Schering et Bayer." *Entreprises et histoire*. N° Spécial: "Industries du médicament et du vivant."

Gerber, Elaine. 2002. "Deconstructing Pregnancy: RU486, Seeing 'Eggs,' and the Ambiguity of Very Early Conceptions." *Medical Anthropology Quarterly* 16 (1): 92–108.

Gillison, Gillian. 1993. *Between Culture and Fantasy: A New Guinea Highlands Mythology*. Chicago: University of Chicago Press.

Ginsburg, Faye, and Rayna Rapp. 1995. *Conceiving the New World Order: The Global Politics of Reproduction*. Berkeley: California University Press.

Gladwell, Malcolm. 2000. "John Rock's Error: What the Co-inventor of the Pill Didn't Know: Menstruation Can Endanger Women's Health." Accessed September 16, 2015. *New Yorker*, March 10. http://gladwell.com/john-rock-s-error/.

Godelier, Maurice. [1982] 1996. *La production des grands hommes: Pouvoir et domination masculine chez les Baruya de Nouvelle-Guinée*. Paris: Flammarion.

Goldenberg, Mirian, org. 2002. *Nu & Vestido. Dez Antropólogos revelam a cultura do corpo carioca*. Rio de Janeiro: Editora Record.

Goldstein, Donna. 2003. *Laughter Out of Place: Race, Class, Violence and Sexuality in a Rio Shantytown*. Berkeley: University of California Press.

Gonçalves, H., A. D. Souza, P. A. Tavares, S. H. Cruz, and D. P. Béhague. 2011. "Contraceptive Medicalisation, Fear of Infertility and Teenage Pregnancy in Brazil." *Culture, Health and Sexuality* 13 (2): 201–15.

Gossel, Patricia Peck. 1999. "Packaging the Pill." In *Manifesting Medicine: Bodies and Machines. Artefacts, Studies in the History of Science and Technology*. Vol. 1. Edited by R. Bud, B. Finn, and H. Trischler, 105–22. Amsterdam: Harwood Academic Publishers.

Greene, Jeremy. 2011. "The Substance of the Brand." *Lancet* 378 (9786): 120–21.

Greene, Raymond, and Katharina Dalton. 1953. "The Premenstrual Syndrome." *British Medical Journal* 1, no. 4818 (May 9): 1007–14.

Greenslit, Nathan. 2005. "Depression and Consumption: Psychopharmaceuticals, Branding, and New Identity Practices." *Culture, Medicine and Psychiatry* 29 (4): 477–501.

Gregor, Thomas, and Donald Tuzun. 2001. *Gender in Amazonia and Melanesia*. Berkeley, University of California Press.

Grosz, Elizabeth. 1994. *Volatile Bodies: Toward a Corporeal Feminism*. Bloomington: Indiana University Press.

Guedes, Alessandra. 2000. "Abortion in Brazil: Legislation, Reality and Options." *Reproductive Health Matters* 8 (16): 66–76.

Guterman, M. A. 2006. "Identity Conflict in Modern Orthodox Judaism and the Laws of Family Purity." *Method and Theory in the Study of Religion* 18 (1): 92–100.

Hacking, Ian. 2007. "Kinds of People: Moving Targets." *Proceedings of the British Academy* 151: 285–318.

Haraway, Donna. 2008. *When Species Meet*. Posthumanities, Vol. 3. Minneapolis: University of Minnesota Press.

Haraway, Donna. 2004. "A Manifesto for Cyborgs: Science, Technology, and Socialist Feminism in the 1980s." In *The Haraway Reader*, 7–46. New York: Routledge.

Haraway, Donna. 1997. *Modest_Witness@Second_Millennium.FemaleMan©_Meets_Onco-Mouse™*. London: Routledge.

Haraway, Donna. 1992. "The Promises of Monsters: A Regenerative Politics for Inappropriate/d Others." In *Cultural Studies*, edited by Lawrence Grossberg, Cary Nelson, and Paula Treichler, 295–337. New York: Routledge.

Haraway, Donna. 1991. *Simians, Cyborgs, and Women: The Reinvention of Nature*. New York: Routledge.

Haraway, Donna. 1989. *Primate Visions: Gender, Race and Nature in the World of Modern Science*. New York: Routledge.

Hardon, Anita. 2006. "Contesting Contraceptive Innovation — Reinventing the Script." *Social Science and Medicine* (62): 614–27.

Hartmann, Betsy. 1995. *Reproductive Rights and Wrongs: The Global Politics of Population Control*. Boston: South End Press.

Hayden, Cori. 2013. "Distinctively Similar: A Generic Problem." UC *Davis Law Review* 47 (2): 601–32.

Hayden, Cori. 2007. "A Generic Solution? Pharmaceuticals and the Politics of the Similar in Mexico." *Current Anthropology* 48 (4): 475–95.

Hayward, Eva. 2010. "Spider City Sex." *Women and Performance: A Journal of Feminist Theory* 20 (3): 225–51.

Heilborn, Maria Luiza, Estela Aquino, Michel Bozon, and Daniela Knauth. 2006. *O aprendizado da sexualidade reprodução e trajetórias sociais de jovens brasileiros*. Rio de Janeiro: Editora Fiocruz.

Heilborn, Maria Luiza, Estela Aquino, and Daniela Knauth. 2006. "Juventude, sexualidade e reprodução." *Cadernos de Saúde Pública* 22 (7): 1362–64.

Heilborn, Maria Luiza, and Cristiane da Silva Cabral. 2013. "Youth, Gender and Sexual Practices in Brazil." *Psicologia & Sociedade* 25: 33–43.

Helmreich, Stefan. 2011. "What Was Life? Answers from Three Limit Biologies." *Critical Inquiry* 37 (4): 671–96.

Henare, A., M. Holbraad, and S. Wastell, eds. 2007. *Thinking Through Things: Theorising Artefacts Ethnographically*. London: Routledge.

Héritier, Françoise. 1996. *Masculin/Féminin: La pensée de la différence*. Paris: Odile Jacob.

Heyes, Cressida. 2007. *Self-Transformations: Foucault, Ethics, and Normalized Bodies*. Oxford: Oxford University Press.

Hird, Myra. 2009. "Feminist Engagements with Matter." *Feminist Studies* 35 (2): 329–46.

Hoberman, John. 2005. *Testosterone Dreams: Rejuvenation, Aphrodisia, Doping*. Berkeley: University of California Press.

Holston, James. 2008. *Insurgent Citizenship: Disjunctions of Democracy and Modernity in Brazil*. Princeton, NJ: Princeton University Press.

Holston, James. 1989. *The Modernist City: An Anthropological Critique of Brasília*. Chicago: Chicago University Press.

Idhe, Don. 2000. "Epistemology Engines." *Nature* 406 (6791): 21.

Illich, Ivan. 1976. *Medical Nemesis: The Expropriation of Health*. New York: Pantheon Books.

Ingold, Tim. 2012. "Toward an Ecology of Materials." *Annual Review of Anthropology* 41: 427–42.

Ingold, Tim. 2010. "Bringing Things to Life: Creative Entanglements in a World of Materials." Working Paper no. 15. Manchester: ESRC National Centre for Research Methods.

Ingold, Tim. 2007. "Materials against Materiality." *Archaeological Dialogues* 14 (1): 1–16.

Isley, Michelle M., and Andrew M. Kaunitz. 2011. "Update on Hormonal Contraception and Bone Density." *Reviews in Endocrine and Metabolic Disorders* 12 (2): 93–106.

Johnston-Robledo, Ingrid, Jessica Barnack, and Stephanie Wares. 2006. "'Kiss Your Period Good-Bye': Menstrual Suppression in the Popular Press." *Sex Roles* 54, nos. 5–6: 353–60.

Jones, L. 2011. "Anthropological Fantasies in the Debate over Cycle-Stopping Contraception." *Women's Studies: An Inter-disciplinary Journal* 40 (2): 127–48.

Kaler, Amy. 1998. "A Threat to the Nation and a Threat to the Men: The Banning of Depo-Provera in Zimbabwe, 1981." *Journal of Southern African Studies* 24 (2): 347–76.

Kirksey, Eben. 2014. *The Multispecies Salon*. Durham, NC: Duke University Press.

Kissling, E. A. 2013. "Pills, Periods, and Postfeminism." *Feminist Media Studies* 13 (3): 490–504.

Kissling, Elizabeth. 2006. *Capitalizing on the Curse: The Business of Menstruation*. Boulder, CO: Lynne Rienner.

Knight, Chris. 1991. *Blood Relations: Menstruation and the Origins of Culture*. New Haven, CT: Yale University Press.

Konrad, Monica. 1998. "Ova Donation and Symbols of Substance: Some Variations on the Theme of Sex, Gender and the Partible Body." *Journal of the Royal Anthropological Institute* 4 (4): 643–67.

Kristeva, Julia. 1982. *Powers of Horror: An Essay on Abjection*, translated by Leon S. Roudiez. New York: Columbia University Press.

Kulick, Don. 1998. *Travesti: Sex, Gender, and Culture among Brazilian Transgendered Prostitutes*. Chicago: University of Chicago Press.

Lagrou, Els. 2007. *A fluidez da forma: arte, alteridade e agência emu ma sociedade amazônica (Kaxinawa, Acre)*. Rio de Janeiro: TopBoks Editora.

Landecker, Hannah, and Aaron Panofsky. 2013. "From Social Structure to Gene Regulation, and Back: A Critical Introduction to Environmental Epigenetics for Sociology." *Annual Review of Sociology* 39: 333–57.

Laqueur, Thomas. 2003. "Sex in the Flesh: Reply." *Isis* 94: 300–306.

Laqueur, Thomas. 1990. *Making Sex: Body and Gender from the Greeks to Freud*. Cambridge, MA: Harvard University Press.

Latour, Bruno. 2011. "A Cautious Prometheus? A Few Steps Toward a Philosophy of Design with Special Attention to Peter Sloterdijk." In *In Medias Res: Peter Sloterdijk's*

Spherological Poetics of Being, edited by Willem Schinkel and Liesbeth Noordegraaf-Eelens, 151–64. Amsterdam: Amsterdam University Press.

Latour, Bruno. 2004. "Why Has Critique Run Out of Steam? From Matters of Fact to Matters of Concern." *Critical Inquiry* 30 (2): 225–48.

Latour, Bruno. 1999. *Pandora's Hope: Essays on the Reality of Science Studies*. Cambridge, MA: Harvard University Press.

Laws, Sophie, Valerie Hey, and Andrea Eagan. 1985. *Seeing Red: The Politics of Premenstrual Tension*. London: Hutchinson.

Leal, Ondina Fachel. 1995. "Sangue, Fertilidade e Práticas Conraceptivas." In *Corpo e Significado: Ensaios de Antropologia Social*, edited by O. F. Leal. Porto Alegre: NUPACS, Editora da Universidade Federal do Rio Grande do Sul.

Leal, Ondina Fachel, and Bernardo Lewgoy. 1995. "Pessoa, Aborto e Contracepção." *Corpo e Significado: Ensaios de Antropologia Social*, edited by O. F. Leal. Porto Alegre: NUPACS, Editora da Universidade Federal do Rio Grande do Sul.

Leder, Drew. 1990. *The Absent Body*. Chicago: Chicago University Press.

Lévi-Strauss, Claude. 1981. *The Naked Man: Mythologiques*, vol. 4. Chicago: Chicago University Press.

Lewis, Gilbert. 1988. *Day of Shining Red: An Essay on Understanding Ritual*. Cambridge: Cambridge University Press.

Leys, Ruth. 2011. "On Catherine Malabou's What Should We Do With Our Brain?" *nonsite.org* (2). Accessed June 12, 2014. http://nonsite.org/issues/issue-2/on-catherine -malabous-what-should-we-do-with-our-brain.

Lima, T. 2005. *Um peixe olhou para mim: o povo Yudjá e a perspectiva*. 1st ed. São Paulo: ISA/ Editora Unesp/NuTI.

Livingstone, Julie. 2012. *Improvising Medicine: An African Cancer Ward in an Emerging Cancer Epidemic*. Durham, NC: Duke University Press.

Lock, Margaret. 1993. *Encounters with Ageing: Mythologies of Menopause in Japan and North America*. Berkeley: University of California Press.

Lock, Margaret, and Judith Farquhar, eds. 2007. *Beyond the Body Proper: Reading the Anthropology of Material Life*. Durham, NC: Duke University Press.

Lovell, Anne. 2013. "Elusive Travelers: Russian Narcology, Transnational Toxicomanias, and the Great French Ecological Experiment." In *Addiction Trajectories*, edited by Eugene Raikhel and William Garriott, 126–59. Durham, NC: Duke University Press.

Lovell, Anne. 2006. "Addiction Markets: The Case of High-Dose Buprenorphine in France." In *Global Pharmaceuticals: Ethics, Markets, Practices*, edited by Adriana Petryna, Andrew Lakoff, and Arthur Kleinman, 136–70. Durham, NC: Duke University Press.

Löwy, Ilana. 2013. "Treating Health Risks or Putting Healthy Women at Risk: Controversies around Chemoprevention of Breast Cancer." In *Ways of Regulating Drugs in the 19th and 20th Centuries*, edited by Jean-Paul Gaudilliere and Volker Hess, 206–27. Houndmills, UK: Palgrave Macmillan.

Löwy, Ilana. 2012. "Cancer du sein et tamoxifène: Gestion d'une incertitude thérapeutique." *Sciences Sociales et Santé* 30 (1): 73–83.

Löwy, Ilana, and George Weisz. 2005. "French Hormones: Progestins and Therapeutic Variation in France." *Social Science and Medicine* 60 (11): 2609–22.

Loyola, Maria Andrea. 2010. "Cinquenta anos de anticoncepção hormonal: a mulher e a pílula." *ComCiência*, no. 119.

MacDonald, Paul, Raymond Dombroski, and Linette Casey. 1991. "Recurrent Secretion of Progesterone in Large Amounts: An Endocrine/Metabolic Disorder Unique to Young Women? *Endocrine Reviews* 12 (4): 372–401.

Makuch, M. Y., M. J. D. Osis, K. S. de Pádua, and L. Bahamondes. 2013. "Use of Hormonal Contraceptives to Control Menstrual Bleeding: Attitudes and Practice of Brazilian Gynecologists." *International Journal of Women's Health* 5: 795–801.

Malabou, Catherine. 2011. *Que faire de notre cerveau?* Paris: Éditions Bayard.

Malysse, Stéphane. 2002. Em busca dos (H)alteres-ego: Olhares frances nos bastidores da corpolatria carioca. In *Nu & Vestido. Dez Antropólogos revelam a cultura do corpo carioca*, org. Goldenberg, Mirian. Rio de Janeiro: Editora Record.

Mamo, L., and J. R. Fosket. 2009. "Scripting the Body: Pharmaceuticals and the (re)making of Menstruation." *Signs: Journal of Women in Culture and Society* 34 (4): 925–49.

Manica, Daniela. 2011. "A desnaturalização da menstruação: Hormônios contraceptivos e tecnociência." *Horizontes Antropológicos* 17 (35): 197–226.

Manica, Daniela. 2009. *Contracepção, natureza e cultura: Embates e sentidos na etnografia de uma trajetória*. Tese (Doutorado em Antropologia Social). Campinas: Instituto de Filosofia e Ciências Humanas, Universidade Estadual de Campinas.

Marcus, George. 1995 [1998]. "Ethnography in/of the World System: The Emergence of Multi-sited Ethnography." In *Ethnography Through Thick and Thin*. Princeton, NJ: Princeton University Press.

Marinho, Lilian, Estela Aquino, and Conceição Almeida. 2009. "Contraceptive Practices and Sexual Initiation among Young People in Brazil." *Cadernos e Saúde Pública* 25 (Suppl. 2): S227–39.

Marks, Lara. 2001. *Sexual Chemistry: A History of the Contraceptive Pill*. New Haven, CT: Yale University Press.

Martin, Emily. 2006. "The Pharmaceutical Person." *BioSocieties* 1 (3): 273–87.

Martin, Emily. [1987] 2001. *The Woman in the Body: A Cultural Analysis of Reproduction*. 3rd ed. Boston: Beacon Press.

Martin, Emily. 1994. *Flexible Bodies: The Role of Immunity in American Culture from the Days of Polio to the Age of AIDS*. Boston: Beacon Press.

Martins, Poliana Cardoso, Rosangela Minardi Mitre Cotta, Fábio Farias Mendes, Sylvia do Carmo Castro Franceschinni, Silvia Eloiza Priore, Glauce Dias, and Rodrigo Siqueira-Batista. 2008. "Conselhos de saúde e a participação social no Brasil: Matizes da utopia." *Physis* 18 (1): 105–21.

Masco, J. 2013. "Side Effect." *Somatosphere*. Accessed January 22, 2015. http://somatosphere.net/2013/12/side-effect.html.

McCallum, Cecilia. 2014. "Cashinahua Perspectives on Functional Anatomy: Ontology, Ontogenesis, and Biomedical Education in Amazonia." *American Ethnologist* 41: 504–17.

McCallum, Cecilia. 2005a. "Explaining Caesarean Section in Salvador da Bahia, Brazil." *Sociology of Health and Illness* 27 (2): 215–42.

McCallum, Cecilia. 2005b. "Racialized Bodies, Naturalized Classes: Moving Through the City of Salvador da Bahia." *American Ethnologist* 32 (1): 100–117.

McCallum, Cecilia, and Ana Paula dos Reis. 2008. "Users' and Carers' Perspectives on Technological Procedures for 'Normal' Childbirth in a Public Maternity Hospital in Salvador, Brazil." *Salud Publico México* 50 (1): 40–48.

McGoey, Linsey. 2012. "Strategic Unknowns: Towards a Sociology of Ignorance." *Economy and Society* 41 (1): 1–16.

Mello, João Cardoso de, and Fernando Novais. 1998. "Capitalismo Tardio e Sociabilidade Moderna." In *História da Vida Privada no Brasil*. Vol. 4. *Contrastes da Intimidade Contemporânea*. Edited by Lilia Moritz Schwarcz. São Paulo: Companhia das Letras.

Mendes, Eugênio. 1996. O sistema único de saúde: Um processo social em construção. In *Uma agenda para a saúde*, org. Eugênio Mendes, 57–98. São Paulo: Hucitec.

Menezes, Greice, and Estela Aquino. 2009. "Pesquisa sobre o aborto no Brasil: Avanços e desafios para o campo da saúde coletiva." *Cadernos de Saúde Pública* 25: S193–204.

Menezes, Greice, Estela Aquino, and Diorlene Oliveira da Silva. 2006. "Induced Abortion during Youth: Social Inequalities in the Outcome of the First Pregnancy." *Cadernos de Saúde Pública* 22 (7): 1431–46.

Mintzes, Barbara, Anita Hardon, and Jannemieke Hanhart. 1993. *Norplant: Under Her Skin.* Amsterdam: Eburon for Women's Health Action Foundation and WEMOS.

Moerman, Daniel. 2002. *Meaning, Medicine and the "Placebo Effect."* Cambridge: Cambridge University Press.

Mol, Annemarie. 2013. "Mind your plate! The Ontonorms of Dutch Dieting." *Social Studies of Science* 43 (3): 379–96.

Mol, Annemarie. 2008. *The Logic of Care: Health and the Problem of Patient Choice.* London: Routledge.

Mol, Annemarie. 2002. *The Body Multiple: Ontology in Medical Practice.* Durham, NC: Duke University Press.

Montgomery, Rita. 1974. "A Cross-Cultural Study of Menstruation, Menstrual Taboos, and Related Social Variables." *Ethos* 2 (2): 137–70.

Mosko, Mark. 1985. *Quadripartite Structures: Categories, Relations and Homologies in Bush Mekeo Culture.* Cambridge: Cambridge University Press.

Murphy, Michelle. 2012. *Seizing the Means of Reproduction: Entanglements of Feminism, Health, and Technoscience.* Durham, NC: Duke University Press.

Murphy, Michelle. 2011. "Distributed Reproduction." In *Corpus: Bodies of Knowledge*, edited by Paisley Currah and Monica Casper, 21–38. New York: Palgrave Macmillan.

Murphy, Michelle. 2008. "Chemical Regimes of Living." *Environmental History* 13 (4): 695–703.

Nading, Alex. 2014. "Global Health and Its Things: Thoughts on Becoming with Chemicals That Kill." Paper presented at the Embodied Being, Environing World: Local Biologies and Local Ecologies in Global Health Workshop. Paris, June 5–6. Collège d'études mondiales, FMSH, IEA.

Natansohn, Graciela. 2005. "O Corpo Feminino como objeto médico e 'mediatico.'" *Revista Estudos Feministas* 13 (2): 287–305.

Oldani, M. 2004. Thick Prescriptions: Toward an Interpretation of Pharmaceutical Sales Practices. *Medical Anthropology Quarterly* 18: 325–56.

Oudshoorn, Nelly. 1997. "From Population Control Politics to Chemicals: The WHO as an Intermediary Organization in Contraceptive Development." *Social Studies of Science* 27 (1): 41–72.

Oudshoorn, Nelly. 1996. "The Decline of the One-Size-Fits-All Paradigm, or, How Reproductive Scientists Try to Cope with Postmodernity." In *Monsters, Goddesses and Cyborgs: Feminist Confrontations with Science, Medicine and Cyberspace*, edited by Nina Lykke and Rosi Braidotti, 153–72. London: Zed Books.

Oudshoorn, Nelly. 1994. *Beyond the Natural Body: an archeology of sex hormones*. London: Routledge.

Padua, K. S., M. J. Osis, A. Faundes, A. H. Barbosa, and O. B. Moraes Filho. 2010. "Factors Associated with Cesarean Sections in Brazilian Hospitals." *Revista de Saúde Pública* 44 (1): 70–79.

Pallavi, Aparna. 2005. "Purity at a Price." *Financial Daily*. Accessed December 13, 2007. http://www.thehindubusinessline.com/life/2005/10/28/stories/2005102800090200.htm.

Parés, Luis Nicolau. 2006. *A formação do Candomblé: História e ritual da nação jeje na Bahia*. Campinas: Editora Unicamp.

Parker, Richard. 1991. *Bodies, Pleasures, and Passions: Sexual Culture in Contemporary Brazil*. Boston: Beacon Press.

Pedro, Joana Maria. 2003. "A experiência com contraceptivos no Brasil: Uma questão de geração." *Revista Brasileira de História* 23 (45): 239–60.

Perpétuo, Ignez, and Laura Wong. 2009. "Desigualdade socioeconômica na utilização de métodos anticoncepcionais no Brasil." In *Pesquisa Nacional de Demografia e Saúde: Dimensões do Processo Reprodutivo e da Saúde da Criança*. Ministério da Saúde, Brasília: Centro Brasileiro de Análise e Planejamento.

Pert, Candace. [1997] 2003. *The Molecules of Emotion: The Science behind Mind-Body Medicine*. New York: Scribner.

Peterson, Kristin. 2014. *Speculative Markets: Drug Circuits and Derivative Life in Nigeria*. Durham, NC: Duke University Press.

Petryna, Adriana. 2009. "Pharmaceuticals and the Right to Health." In *When Experiments Travel: Clinical Trials and the Global Search for Human Subjects*, 139–86. Princeton, NJ: Princeton University Press.

Petryna, Adriana, Andrew Lakoff, and Arthur Kleinman, eds. 2006. *Global Pharmaceuticals: Ethics, Markets, Practices*. Durham, NC: Duke University Press.

Pinheiro-Machado, Rosana, and Alexander S. Dent. 2013. "Paradoxes of Development: Why Now?" *Fieldsights—Hot Spots, Cultural Anthropology Online*. Accessed July 20, 2015. http://culanth.org/fieldsights/444-paradoxes-of-development-why-now.

Pompei, L. M., C. E. Fernandes, M. L. Steiner, R. Strufaldi, and N. R. Melo. 2013. "Attitudes, Knowledge and Prescribing Habits of Brazilian Gynecologists Regarding Extended-Cycle Oral Contraceptives." *Gynecological Endocrinology* 29 (12): 1071–74.

Pordié, Laurent, and Jean-Paul Gaudillière. 2014. "The Reformulation Regime in Drug Discovery: Revisiting Polyherbals and Property Rights in the Ayurvedic Industry." *East Asian Science, Technology and Society: An International Journal* 8: 57–79.

Pottage, Alain. 1998. "Power as an Art of Contingency: Luhmann, Deleuze, Foucault." *Economy and Society* 27 (1): 1–27.

Pouchelle, Marie-Christine. 2008. "Humeurs corporelles à l'hôpital." Presentation given at the "Humeurs et Dégoûts: Du dispositive à l'institution" workshop, January 16, 2008, Maison des sciences de l'Homme, Paris.

Prior, Jerilynn, and Christine Hitchcock. 2014. "Manipulating Menstruation with Hormonal Contraception: What Does the Science say?" Centre for Menstrual Cycle and Ovulation Research. Accessed September 16, 2015. http://www.cemcor.ubc.ca/resources/manipulating-menstruation-hormonal-contraception—what-does-science-say.

Proctor, Robert, and Londa Schiebinger. 2008. *Agnotology. The Making and Unmaking of Ignorance.* Stanford, CA: Stanford University Press.

Rabinow, Paul. 1996. "Artificiality and Enlightenment: From Sociobiology to Biosociality." In *Essays on the Anthropology of Reason*, 91–111. Princeton, NJ: Princeton University Press.

Rabinow, Paul, and Nikolas Rose. 2006. "Biopower Today." *BioSocieties* 1: 195–217.

Rapp, Rayna. 2000. *Testing Women, Testing the Fetus: The Social Impact of Amniocentesis in America.* New York: Routledge.

Rebhun, Linda. 1993. "Nerves and Emotional Play in Northeast Brazil." *Medical Anthropology Quarterly* 7 (2): 131–51.

Reeves Sanday, Peggy. 1981. *Female Power and Male Dominance: On the Origins of Sexual Inequality.* Cambridge: Cambridge University Press.

Ribeiro, Darcy. 1995. *O Povo Brasileiro: A formação e o sentido de Brasil.* 2nd ed. São Paulo: Companhia das Letras.

Roberts, Elizabeth. 2012. *God's Laboratory: Assisted Reproduction in the Andes.* Berkeley: University of California Press.

Roberts, Elizabeth. 2008. "Biology, Sociality and Reproductive Modernity in an Ecuadorian In-vitro Fertilization: The Particulars of Place." In *Biosocialities, Genetics and the Social Sciences: Making Biologies and Identities*, edited by Sahra Gibbon and Carlos Novas, 79–97. London: Routledge.

Rohden, Fabíola. 2008. "O império dos hormônios e a construção da diferença entre os sexos." *História, Ciências, Saúde—Manguinhos* 15: 133–52.

Rohden, Fabíola. 2003. *A Arte de Enganar a Natureza: contracepção, aborto e infanticídio no início do século XX.* Rio de Janeiro: Editora Fiocruz.

Rohden, Fabíola. 2001. *Uma Ciência da Diferença: Sexo e gênero na medicina da mulher.* Rio de Janeiro: Editora Fiocruz.

Rose, Nikolas. 2007. *The Politics of Life Itself: Biomedicine, Power, and Subjectivity in the Twenty-First Century.* Princeton, NJ: Princeton University Press.

Rose, Nikolas, and Carlos Novas. 2006. "Biological Citizenship." In *Global Assemblages: Technology, Politics and Ethics as Anthropological Problems*, edited by Aihwa Wong and Stephen J. Collier, 439–63. Oxford: Blackwell.

Rotania, Alejandra. 2000. "Formas atuais de intervenção no corpo das mulheres." In *Mulheres, Corpo e Saúde*, edited by Nalu Faria and Maria Lucia Silveira. São Paulo: Cadernos Sempreviva.

Rozenberg, Riva, Katia Silveira da Silva, Claudia Bonan, and Eloane Gonçalves Ramos. 2013. "Práticas contraceptivas de adolescentes brasileiras: Vulnerabilidade social em questão." *Ciênia & Saúde Coletiva* 18 (12): 3645–52.

Sagan, Dorion, and Lynn Margulis. 1991. "Epilogue: The Uncut Self." In *Organism and the Origins of Self*, edited by Alfred Tauber. Dordrecht, Netherlands: Kluwer Academic Publishers.

Sanabria, E. 2014. "'The Same Thing in a Different Box': Similarity and Difference in Pharmaceutical Sex Hormone Consumption and Marketing." *Medical Anthropology Quarterly* 28 (4): 537–55.

Sanabria, E. 2011. "Pourquoi saigner?" *Terrain: Analyses de sang* (56): 42–57.

Sanabria, E. 2010. "Le médicament, un objet évanescent : Essai sur la fabrication et la consommation des substances pharmaceutiques." *Techniques and Culture*, nos. 52–53: 168–89.

Sanabria, E. 2009. "Alleviative Bleeding: Bloodletting, Menstruation and the Politics of Ignorance in a Brazilian Blood Donation Centre." *Body and Society* 15 (2): 123–44.

Sansone, Livio. 2003. *Blackness without Ethnicity: Constructing Race in Brazil*. Houndmills, UK: Palgrave Macmillan.

Santow, Gigi. 2001. "Emmenagogues and Abortifacients in the Twentieth Century: An Issue of Ambiguity." In *Regulating Menstruation: Beliefs, Practices, and Interpretations*, edited by Etienne van de Walle and Elisha Renne, 64–92. Chicago: University of Chicago Press.

Scheper-Hughes, Nancy. 1992. *Death without Weeping: The Violence of Everyday Life in Brazil*. Berkeley: University of California Press.

Schneider, D. M. [1968] 1980. *American Kinship: A Cultural Account*. Chicago: University of Chicago Press.

Shuttle, Penelope, and Peter Redgrove. 1978. *The Wise Wound: Menstruation and Everywoman*. London: Marion Boyars.

Snow, Loudell. [1993] 1998. *Walkin' Over Medicine*. Detroit: Wayne State University Press.

Snow, Rachel, Ellen Hardy, Elsbeth Kneuper, Eliana Hebling, and Grace Halla. 2007. "Women's Responses to Menses and Nonbleeding Intervals in the USA, Brazil and Germany." *Contraception* 76: 23–29.

Soto Laveaga, Gabriela. 2009. *Jungle Laboratories: Mexican Peasants, National Projects, and the Making of the Pill*. Durham, NC: Duke University Press.

Spitzer, W. O. 1997. "The 1995 Pill Scare Revisited: Anatomy of a Non-epidemic." *Human Reproduction* 12 (11): 2347–57.

Stegeman, B. H., M. deBastos, F. R. Rosendaal, A. van Hylckama Vlieg, F. M. Helmerhorst, T. Stijnen, and O. M. Dekkers. 2013. "Different Combined Oral Contraceptives and the Risk of Venous Thrombosis: Systematic Review and Network Meta-analysis." *BMJ* 347: f5298.

Stengers, Isabelle. 2014. "Penser à partir du ravage écologique." *De l'univers clos au monde infini*, edited by E. Hache. Paris: Éditions Dehors.

Strassmann, Beverly. 1997. "The Biology of Menstruation in Homo sapiens: Total Lifetime Menses, Fecundity, and Nonsynchrony in a Natural-Fertility Population." *Current Anthropology* 38 (1): 123–29.

Strathern, Marilyn. 2004. "The Whole Person and Its Artifacts." *Annual Review of Anthropology* 33: 1–19.

Strathern, Marilyn. 1992a. *After Nature: English Kinship in the Late Twentieth Century*. Cambridge: Cambridge University Press.

Strathern, Marilyn. 1992b. *Reproducing the Future: Essays on Anthropology, Kinship and the New Reproductive Technologies*. Manchester, UK: Manchester University Press.

Strathern, Marilyn. 1991. *Partial Connections*. Lanham, MD: Rowman and Littlefield.

Strathern, Marilyn. 1988. *The Gender of the Gift: Problems with Women and Problems with Society in Melanesia*. Berkeley: University of California Press.

Sunder Rajan, Kaushik. Forthcoming. "Pharmocracy: Trials of Global Biomedicine." Durham, NC: Duke University Press.

Sunder Rajan, Kaushik, ed. 2012. *Lively Capital: Biotechnologies, Ethics, and Governance in Global Markets*. Durham, NC: Luke University Press.

Taussig, Michael. 2012. *Beauty and the Beast*. Chicago: University of Chicago Press.

Thomas, Sarah, and Charlotte Ellertson. 2000. "Nuisance or Natural and Healthy: Should Monthly Menstruation Be Optional for Women?" *Lancet* 355 (9207): 922–24.

Tone, Andrea. 2001. *Devices and Desires: A History of Contraceptives in America*. New York: Hill and Wang.

United Nations Population Fund. 1999. *The UNFPA Private-Sector Initiative. Exploring Ways to Facilitate Cooperation Between Governments and the Commercial Sector to Expand Access to Reproductive Health Commodities*. Issue 48 of Technical Report. New York: UNFPA.

Van de Port, Mattijs. 2012. "Genuinely Made Up: Camp, Baroque, and Other Denaturalizing Aesthetics in the Cultural Production of The Real." *Journal of the Royal Anthropological Institute* 18 (4): 864–83.

Van de Port, Mattijs. 2011. *Ecstatic Encounters: Bahian Candomblé and the Quest for the Really Real*. Amsterdam: Amsterdam University Press.

van der Geest, S., S. R. Whyte, and A. Hardon. 1996. "The Anthropology of Pharmaceuticals: A Biographical Approach." *Annual Review of Anthropology* 25: 153–78.

van de Walle, Etienne, and Elisha Renne. 2001. *Regulating Menstruation: Beliefs, Practices, and Interpretations*. Chicago: University of Chicago Press.

Victora, Cesar, Estela Aquino, Maria do Carmo Leal, Carolos Monteiro, Fernando Barros, and Celia Szwarcwald. 2011. "Maternal and Child Health in Brazil: Progress and Challenges." *Lancet* 377 (9780): 1863–76.

Vigarello, Georges. 2004. *Histoire de la beauté, corps et embellissement de la renaissance à nos jours*. Paris: Seuil.

Vilaça, Aparecida. 2005. "Chronically Unstable Bodies: Reflections on Amazonian Corporalities." *Journal of the Royal Anthropological Institute* 11 (3): 445–64.

Viveiros de Castro, Eduardo. 2012. "Cosmological Perspectivism in Amazonia and Elsewhere." Masterclass Series. Vol. 1. Manchester, UK: *Hau* Network of Ethnographic Theory.

Viveiros de Castro, Eduardo. 2007a. "O perspectivismo é a retomada da Antropofagia oswaldiana em novos termos." In *Encontros: Eduardo Viveiros de Castro*, edited by Renato Sztutman. Rio de Janeiro: Beco do Azougue Editorial Ltda.

Viveiros de Castro, Eduardo. 2007b. *Transversal Shamanism. Form and Force in Amazonian Cosmopolitics.* Paper presented at the Senior Seminar, Department of Social Anthropology, University of Cambridge.

Viveiros de Castro, Eduardo, and Marcio Goldman. 2012. "Introduction to Post-Social Anthropology Networks, Multiplicities, and Symmetrizations." HAU: *Journal of Ethnographic Theory* 2 (1): 421–33.

Walker, Anne. 1995. "Theory and Methodology in Premenstrual Syndrome Research." *Social Science and Medicine* 41 (6): 793–800.

Watkins, Elizabeth. 2012. "How the Pill Became a Lifestyle Drug: The Pharmaceutical Industry and Birth Control in the United States Since 1960." *American Journal of Public Health* 102 (8): 1462–72.

Weiner, James. 1995. *The Lost Drum: The Myth of Sexuality in Papua New Guinea and Beyond.* Madison: University of Wisconsin Press.

Weismantel, Mary. 2001. *Cholas and Pishtacos: Stories of Race and Sex in the Andes.* Chicago: University of Chicago Press.

Weismantel, Mary, and Stephen F. Eisenman. 1998. "Race in the Andes: Global Movements and Popular Ontologies." *Bulletin for Latin American Research* 17: 121–42.

Weston, K. 1995. "Forever Is a Long Time: Romancing the Real in Gay Kinship Ideologies." In *Naturalizing Power: Essays in Feminist Cultural Analysis*, edited by S. Yanagisako and C. Delaney, 87–110. New York: Routledge.

Whyte, Susan, R. Sjaak van der Geest, and Anita Hardon. 2002. *Social Lives of Medicines.* Cambridge: Cambridge University Press.

Winant, Howard. 1992. "Rethinking Race in Brazil." *Journal of Latin American Studies* 24: 173–92.

Yates-Doerr, Emily. 2015. "Intervals of Confidence: Uncertain Accounts of Hunger, Weight, and Global Health." *Biosocieties* 10: 227–46.

Yates-Doerr, Emily. 2014. "The World in a Box? Food Security, Edible Insects, and 'One World, One Health' Collaboration." *Social Science and Medicine* 129: 106–12.

Zimmerman, Deena. 2012. "Hormonal Cycle Manipulation." *Jewish Women's Health: The Hilchot Niddah Guide for Medical Professionals.* NISHMAT Centre for Advanced Torah Study for Women. Accessed April 16, 2014. http://www.jewishwomenshealth.org/print.php?article=74.

Žižek, Slavoj. 2006. *The Parallax View.* Cambridge, MA: MIT Press.

Zuk, Marlene. 2013. *Paleofantasy: What Evolution Really Tells Us about Sex, Diet, and How We Live.* New York: W. W. Norton.

INDEX

Page numbers followed by *f* indicate illustrations; page numbers followed by t indicate tables.

Beltrán, Carlos López, 36
Berenstein, Elizer, 168
Biehl, João, 133, 150–51
bioavailability, 132, 153–55, 168, 180, 182–83
biomedical regimes: and access to medical services, 129–30; and class, 151
biopolitics, 5, 131, 149–50, 190; and democratization, 155–58; and plasticity, 199–201
birth: and blood, 59–60; natural versus cesarean, 7, 151; and status hierarchies, 35
birth rates, 75–76, 133
blood: birth blood, 30–31; hormônio compared to, 107–8, 118–23; and implants, 86; and the pill, 95; and racial categories, 36; sangue, 118–19; as substance, 122–23, 214–15n15, 216n10. See also menstrual blood
blood donation, 21, 118, 120, 121
bloodletting, 92, 118
blood pressure, measuring of, 27
Boa Forma (magazine), 173
bodies, interior/exterior of. See boundaries, bodily
Bodies That Matter (Butler), 127–28
bodies/the body: awareness of and menstruation, 44, 86–87; Bahian modes of embodiment, 198–99; boundaries of, 56–57; and class, 33–34, 35–37; exams/management of in Brazil, 27–28; humoral understanding of, 115, 118–19, 121–23; materiality of, 127–28, 198–99; noncyclical as norm, 44, 45–48, 79, 81–82; open/closed, 54–55, 64–65, 99; plasticity of, 6, 101–2, 190–92, 193, 197; public visibility of, 19–20; versus self, 44, 45, 46–47, 48, 66, 67, 190–91; separable/inseparable distinction, 94–95; and sex/gender, 127–28; stability/malleability of, 37–39, 101–2; as unbounded, 37–38, 40; women's

knowledge of, 20–21, 160. See also embodiment, modes of; knowledge about the body
bodily dys-appearance, 47, 66, 67–68
Boltanski, Luc, 200, 204
bone density, loss of, 17
boundaries: and intervention, 203; of pharmaceutical objects, 177
boundaries, bodily, 187, 188–89; negotiation of, 56–57, 61–66, 68
Bozon, Michel, 133
bracketing (STS), 107
Brazil: biomedical intervention in, 6–7, 129; cultural identities in, 196, 198; family planning policy in, 133, 135–36; fertility rates in, 133; history of health statistics in, 217–18n11; Salvador da Bahia, 21–22, 25–26, 193–94, 195–96; sexual culture of, 24–25; social hierarchies in, 210n18
Brazilian Gynecological Endocrinology Society (SOBRAGE), 78, 169, 173
Brazilian Society for Endocrinology and Metabolism, 173
breastfeeding/breastmilk, 3, 75, 101, 122, 124, 216n11
breasts, growth of with hormônio, 123–24
Browner, Carole, 95
Brumberg, Joan, 57
Buckley, Thomas, 56
Butler, Judith, 127–28

Caldeira, Teresa, 37–38
Callard, Felicity, 200
cancer: and hormone therapy, 154; and implants, 169; and menstrual suppression, 3, 79; risk of, 17, 208n10; and testosterone, 112
Candomblé, 24, 51, 99–100
cannibalism/anthropophagy, 197–98
capital: beauty as, 36–37; knowledge about the body as, 139–41; plasticity as resistance against, 199–200

care, matters of, 206

Carsten, Janet, 122, 216n10

CEPARH (Centre for Research and Assistance in Human Reproduction), 1; author's access to, 2, 19; at gynecological congresses, 168–69; implant insertions at, 170–72; implants produced by, 14–15t, 145, 165–68; low-income patients at, 2, 141; sterilizations at, 141–44, 218n19

cesarean deliveries, 28–29, 30, 151

chemical arbitrage, 162, 220n3

Chiapello, Eve, 200, 204

chipes da beleza (beauty chips), 171, 173

choice, logic of, 113, 203–4

cholesterol levels, 146, 169–70

Ciclo 21 (oral contraceptive), 14–15t

citizenship: and democratization, 155–57; and drug packaging, 149; and family planning, 138; and molar/molecular biopolitics, 148–50, 154–55; and reproductive health, 132–33

City of Walls (Caldeira), 38

class: and access to abortion, 97–98, 152–53; and access to health care, 29–32, 88, 129–30, 131, 156–57; and bodies, 33–34, 35–37; and cost of sanitary products, 59; criteria for middle class, 210n19; and family planning, 133–35, 138, 140–44; and implants, 145–46; and industrialization, 32–33; and medical knowledge, 116, 138, 140; and medical representations of menstruation, 49–50; and menstrual suppression, 88–90, 145; and modernity, 151–52; and personalization/standardization, 150–54; and PMT, 90–92; and pregnancy, 219n24; and social hierarchies, 210n18

cleansing. See *limpeza* (cleanliness)

cloth pads, 57, 60

coagulos (blood coagulates), 67

Cohen, Lawrence, 153

colonialism, postcolonial relations, 196, 197–98

constructivism, 194–95

consumption, 177–78, 203–4

Contracep (injectible contraceptive), 14–15t, 16f, 132, 135

contraceptive methods: choice of, 61, 211n1; distribution of, 136–37

contraceptives, hormonal: administration methods of, 132, 148–49, 159–61; different forms of, 4, 12; packaging of, 180–81, 182–83; personalization of, 132, 145; prevalence of use of, 4; risk evaluations of, 16–19; as traveling object, 13, 161–62, 177; use of for menstrual suppression, 72; uses of, 174. *See also* implants, hormonal; injections, contraceptive; oral contraceptives

contraceptives, long-acting: and class, 134–35, 148–49; and population control, 12–13

control: hormones as means of self-control, 144–48; menstrual suppression as means of, 68–69, 80–81, 92, 102

corpo aberto (open body), 54–55, 59, 64–65, 99

Corrêa, Marilena, 133

Costa, Jurandir Freire, 33, 219n22

Coutinho, Elsimar, 220n6; author's meeting with, 3, 204; on bloodletting, 92; at Gynecological Endocrinology Congress, 111, 113; on importance of elcometrine, 168; and modeling agencies, 171; on negative effects of menstruation, 78–79; prestige/legitimacy of, 1–2

CRESAR, 136

cuidar-se (self-care), 86–87, 131, 145, 147, 172

Cytotec, 96, 97–98, 213n7

Dalton, Katharina, 79

DaMatta, Roberto, 36–37, 151–52

DATASUS, 137

DeGrandpre, Richard, 13

democratization, 155–58

Depo-Provera (injectible contraceptive), 14–15t, 16f, 132; approval of, 217n6; fibroids treated with, 78; growth of breasts with, 124; interviewees' accounts of, 90, 116–17, 120; marketing of, 134–35; risks of, 17–18, 134, 208n10

design, notion of, 205

desire: and "the real," 193–94

Diniz, Simone, 32, 209n16

dirt. See *limpeza* (cleanliness)

disgust, 62–63

disposição (disposition, desire): lack of due to PMT, 80; maintenance of with hormonal enhancement, 145–46, 147, 174, 182

domestic work, 60

dona do corpo (mistress of the body), 50–51. See also uterus

dos Reis, Ana Paula, 151

Douglas, Mary, 56

"Do You Know Who You Are Talking To?" (DaMatta), 152

drospirenone, 14t, 148, 180–81, 208n9, 220n16

Duarte, Luis Fernando Dias, 68, 91–92

Dumit, Joseph, 28

écart (gap), 199–201. See also nature-artifice distinction

Ecks, Stefan, 132–33

ecstatic corporeality, 47

Ecstatic Encounters (van de Port), 194

Edmonds, Alex, 6, 36, 37

efficacies: different types of, 176–77, 180; production of, 13, 19, 161–63, 169–70, 183, 185; social, 161, 172–73, 176–77; symbolic, 176–77, 180

Eisenman, Stephen F., 35–36

Elaní (extended-regime oral contraceptive), 12f, 14–15t, 220–21n16

elcometrine, 14t, 168, 173

Elmeco (pharmaceutical company), 165, 169

embodiment, modes of: Bahian versus European, 198–99; and menstrual cycle, 44, 45–46, 67–68; and mind-body distinctions, 47–48

emergency contraceptives, 159, 182

emmenagogues, 95–98, 213n8

emotions: and PMT, 80–81, 82–83, 147; public expression of, 48, 83, 84–85

EMS Sigma Farma (pharmaceutical company), 180–81

endocrinology, development of, 105–6

endometriosis, 78–79, 168

EngenderHealth, 28

Enovid (oral contraceptive), 9f, 133, 220n2

environmental effects of hormones, 188–89

estradiol, 14t, 126, 167, 168, 170

estrogen: effects of, 173; importance of, 126

evolutionary rationale for menstrual suppression, 73–76, 101–2

extended-regime pills, 14–15t; in Brazil, 10–11; risks of, 17, 204

Faircloth, Charlotte, 101

family planning, 130–31, 133–36, 137, 141–44, 217n10

farmácias de manipulação (compounding pharmacies), 163–67, 170, 177

Farquhar, Judith, 39

Fausto-Sterling, Anne, 106, 128

Faveret Filho, P., 156

femininity: in Brazilian sexual culture, 25; and medicalization of women's bodies, 37. See also *travestis*

feminism: and depoliticization of health

issues, 32; feminist critical theory, 184–85, 190–91, 195, 206; and over-medicalization of women's bodies, 37

fertility rates, 133, 137

fibroids, uterine: seen as result of *hormônio*, 120–21; treatment of, 77, 78

fibromyalgia, 85

Filho, Hugo Maia, 78

first-pass metabolism, 183, 184

Fitzgerald, Des, 200

flexibility, 40–41, 199–200. *See also* plasticity

A Folha de Sao Paulo, 171

Food and Drug Administration, U.S. (FDA), 3, 17, 220n2

foods: menstrual proscriptions on, 52, 53; and thick blood, 118

Fort, Catherine, 134–35

Foucault, Michel, 149, 199

Frank, Robert, 79, 80

Franklin, Sarah, 102, 192, 216n10

Freyre, Gilberto, 24

Gaudillière, Jean-Paul, 162

gender: and endocrine sex, 106; gender binary and hormone use, 109, 111, 126–27, 128; and hormones, 114, 125–26, 128; and PMT, 91; and sex, 191. *See also* sexual dimorphism; *travestis*

Gender Trouble (Butler), 127

Gestinol 28 (extended-regime oral contraceptive), 14–15t

gestrinone, 14t, 167, 168, 173

Gladwell, Malcolm, 74

Godelier, Maurice, 122

Goldenberg, Mirian, 36

Goldman, Marcio, 39, 196–97

Gottlieb, Alma, 56

Greene, Raymond, 79

Greenslit, Nathan, 175

Gynecological Endocrinology congress (2006), 77–78, 108, 111, 113, 126

gynecological examinations, 61–62, 63–64

gynecologists: and female body knowledge, 160; hormonal contraceptive prescriptions by, 72; patient–doctor relationship, 138–41; and uterine pathologies, 77–79

hair growth, abnormal, 170

Haraway, Donna, 39, 178–79, 193

Hartmann, Betsy, 99

health care, administration of, 136–38

health care, private versus public, 29–32, 129–30, 132–33, 209nn14–15; and democratization, 155, 156–57; and hormonal side effects, 147–48; and personalization/standardization differentiation, 150–52, 154–55; and sterilizations, 141

health education, 57–58

Helmreich, Stefan, 192

Hemoba (blood donation center), 118

Héritier, Françoise, 122

Heyes, Cressida, 190–91

Hitchcock, Christine, 17

HIV/STD Reference Centre of São Paulo, 109

Hoberman, John, 146, 185

Hodge, Ileana, 100

Holston, James, 155–56

hope, moral economy of, 150

hormone replacement therapy, 87–88, 115, 154, 172

hormones: administration methods of, 153–54, 159–61; centrality of in women's health, 4–5; efficacies of, 19, 161–63, 169–70, 172–73, 176–77, 180, 183, 185; environmental effects of, 188–89; interviewees' responses to question about how they work, 116–18; legality of, 173–74; materiality of, 5–6, 128, 161–62, 174–83, 188; packaging

hormones (*continued*)
of, 149, 153, 159–61, 162, 174–75, 182–
83; powdered, 165–67; regulation of,
174–75; and sex/gender distinction,
105–8, 128, 188. See also *hormônio*

hormônio: as fluid/substance, 107–8, 114–
15, 118–19, 122–23; and formation of
growths, 93; meaning of term, 114–15;
travestis' use of, 108–11; women's
views of, 86, 145

humanização (humanization of medical
attention), 29–30, 129–30, 150–51

humor/jokes, 61–62, 138, 139, 140, 141

hygiene. See *limpeza* (cleanliness)

hysterectomies: high rates of, 77; and
menstrual suppression, 94–95; and
religious leaders, 100; and rural
women, 88; women seeking, 120

hysteroscopies, 77

Idhe, Don, 40

ignorancia (ignorance), 116, 138–39,
218n14. *See also* knowledge about the
body

Implanon (subdermal hormonal contraceptive implant), 14–15t, 117, 145, 181

implants, hormonal, 14–15t, 132, 166f,
167f; as alternative to sterilization,
134; as "beauty chips," 171; benefits
of according to retailer, 169–70; and
blood, 86; cost of, 217n3; insertion
of at CEPARH, 170–72; interviewees'
comparisons with oral contraceptives,
86; marketing of, 181; and the pill, 161,
181, 182; in private health system, 145–
46; production of by CEPARH clinic,
165–68; rates of use, 218n20; risks of,
146; swelling from, 87; uses of, 174;
and weight gain/loss, 96, 117, 171,
173

individualized hormones. *See* personalization of biomedical interventions

Ingold, Tim, 40, 161, 178–79

injectable hormones: travestis' preference
for, 108–9

injections, contraceptive, 14–15t, 132;
as alternative to sterilization, 134;
associated with the pill, 161; cost of,
217n3; increase in distribution of,
135; rates of use, 207n5; suggested to
young women, 135; uses of, 174

inside/outside distinction. *See* boundaries, bodily

interventionism, 191–92, 202–4; denun-
ciation of, 37

intrauterine "system." *See* Mirena (intrauterine hormonal contraceptive)

Is Menstruation Obsolete? (Coutinho), 3,
207n3

IUDs (intrauterine devices), 182, 212n12;
and menstrual blood, 61, 62

Jones, Laura, 74–75, 101

knowledge about the body: awareness of
the body, 44, 50–52, 86–87; as capital, 139–41; and class, 116, 138, 140;
ignorancia (ignorance), 116, 138–39,
218n14; and medical regimes, 95, 116,
139; travestis', 116; women's, 20–21, 160

Konrad, Monica, 124–25, 126

Kristeva, Julia, 62–63, 65, 66

Kulick, Don, 123

Lancet, 28

language: about *hormônio*, 114–15; about
menstrual suppression, 204; of cleans-
ing/cleanliness, 53; menstruation described in, 48–49, 78

Laqueur, Thomas, 126–27

Latour, Bruno, 107, 178–79, 205

laundry, management of, 60

leakage, pharmaceutical, 19

leakiness of things, 179–80, 188–89. See
also Ingold, Tim

Leal, Ondina Fachel, 96

Leder, Drew, 47, 51, 67–68, 212n13
Lévi-Strauss, Claude, 94
levonorgestrel, 167, 168, 208n9; fibroids
treated with, 78; in implants, 14t; various administration methods of, 159
Lewgoy, Bernardo, 96
Leys, Ruth, 200–201
Libbs (pharmaceutical company), 14t, 71,
220–21n16
limpeza (cleanliness), 33–34, 53–54,
55–61, 190, 212n7
liver, metabolism by, 183, 184
Lock, Margaret, 39, 76, 185
logic of choice/logic of care tension, 113,
203–4
long-acting reversible contraceptive
methods. See contraceptives, long-
acting
Lovell, Anne, 19

MacDonald, Paul, 73–74, 76
machismo, 25, 83
Malabou, Catherine, 40–41, 205, 222n11;
critiques of, 200–201; on plasticity,
102, 193, 199–200, 202
Malysse, Stéphane, 37
Manica, Daniela, 1
Manifesto antropófago (Andrade), 197–98
marketing of sex hormones, 71, 134–35,
148, 159–61, 180–81, 182–83, 219n1,
219n23
Martin, Emily, 41, 55–56; on assessments of side effects, 16; on language
of menstruation, 49–50, 78; on menstrual management, 59; on PMT, 80,
81–82, 83–84; on self-body relationship, 48
Martins, Poliana Cardoso, 156
Masco, Joseph, 16, 18
masculinity, 25, 83. See also testosterone
mass health, models of, 28
materiality: and consumption, 177–80;
and hormones as objects, 161–62,

174–84, 188; and modes of embodiment, 198–99; objects versus things,
179, 205; and sex, 127–28
McCallum, Cecilia, 28–29, 31, 34–35, 151
medical professionals, 115, 165–67. See
also gynecologists
medical regimes: and access to medical
services, 129–30; and class, 151; and
knowledge about the body, 95, 116, 139
Mello, João Cardoso de, 32, 210n17
men: attitudes toward menstruation,
83, 86; attitudes toward pain, 89; and
family planning, 141–44
menarche, 2, 3, 52
Mendes, Eugênio, 157
Menezes, Greice, 153, 219n24
menopause: discourse around, 76; and
fibroids, 121; and ovaries, 50; and rural
women, 88
menstrual blood: and arterial blood, 119–
20; and bodily boundaries, 57; cleansing properties of, 58, 92–93, 100, 102,
118; in clinical contexts, 61–62, 63–64;
coagulos (blood coagulates), 67; as
dirty, 55, 67; domestic management
of, 58–61; and health, 92; indigenous
views of, 214–15n15; and separable/in-
separable distinction, 94–95; as taboo,
99–100
menstrual cycle: affected by social practices, 189; bodily cues marking stages
of, 45–46, 67; and emotional strength,
81–82; and pill dispensers, 8
menstrual management, 92–98, 102–3;
and abortion, 95–97, 152–53; emmenagogues, 95–98; forms of, 73, 187;
and removal of bodily substances,
93–95; use of term, 73
menstrual suppression: advertising campaign for, 71; and contraception, 93,
181–82; evolutionary rationale for,
73–76, 101–2; as form of menstrual
management, 187, 189–90; gynecolo-

menstrual suppression (*continued*)
gists' prescriptions for, 72; and hysterectomy, 94–95, 120; and ideas about
blood, 119–20; and imagery of menstruation, 78–79; and implants, 145;
interviewees' accounts of, 45; and language of choice, 204; and low-income
women, 88–90; media attention to, 3,
207n3; methods available in Salvador,
14–15t; origins of, 5; PMT as rationale
for, 79–87, 147, 213n6; and population control, 1, 5, 12–13; and pregnancy, 93; and religion, 98–100; and
stability/malleability of bodies, 38; use
of term, 73
menstrual taboos, 55–56, 99–100,
214n13
menstruation: agency granted to, 49; attitudes toward, 43–44; and *corpo aberto*
(open body), 54–55; and embodiment,
44, 45, 67–68; frequency of, 73–74;
language used for, 48–49; lore around,
52–55; medical representations of,
49–50, 78–79; as a modern thing, 2, 3,
73–76, 99, 187, 189–90; narratives of,
48–50; and separable/inseparable distinction, 94–95; sex during, 60
Menstruation: Useless Bleeding (Coutinho),
120
Mesigyna (injectible contraceptive), 16f
Microvlar (oral contraceptive), 14–15t,
120
mind–body distinctions, and embodiment, 47, 67–68
Ministry of Health, 136, 137, 209n14,
213n7, 217n9, 218n11
Mirena (intrauterine hormonal contraceptive), 14–15t, 132, 159; advertising
for, 181; as alternative to sterilization,
134; cost of, 217n3; fibroids treated
with, 78; and the pill, 161, 181–82
miscarriage. See *aborto* (abortion)
misoprostol. See Cytotec

modernity: and class, 151–52, 196; and
menstrual suppression, 102, 145, 187–
88, 190; and nature–artifice distinction, 7; and vaginal versus cesarean
birth, 29, 151
Moerman, Daniel, 176
Mol, Annemarie, 39, 107, 113, 203
molar/molecular biopolitics, 148–50
Montgomery, Malcolm, 6–7, 171, 173,
220n6
motherhood, 25, 75–76, 84, 101. See also
birth; family planning; pregnancy
multiple objects, unity of, 107, 161, 177
Murphy, Michelle, 133, 188, 189

Nading, Alex, 40
Naked Man, The (Lévi-Strauss), 94
National Agency of Supplementary
Health (Brazil), 28
National Meeting of Hormonal Implant
Technologies, 169
natural, the, 192, 193–95, 202–3, 211n23,
214n10
nature–artifice distinction, 3, 101, 189–
92, 193–95, 203; and intervention,
202–3; and miscarriages, 214n10; and
modernization, 7
nervoso, 45, 91–92
Nesterone. See elcometrine
neurobiology, 102, 200–201, 222n11
norethisterone (oral contraceptive), 78,
208n9
Norplant (hormonal implant), 159
Nova (*Cosmopolitan Brasil*), 145
Novais, Fernando, 32, 210n17
Novas, Carlos, 190
Nuvaring (long-acting contraceptive), 4,
160, 181

objecthood. See materiality
Oldani, M., 18, 219n1
Oliveira, P., 156
Oliveira, Raica, 171

one-sex world, 126–27

ontology, 39, 184

optimization of the self, 145–46, 150, 202, 205

oral contraceptives: and artificial menstruation, 3, 8–10, 189; availability of, 14–15t, 132, 135; compared with nonoral, 86, 181–83; development of, 8–12; Elaní, 12f, 14–15t, 220–21n16; Enovid, 9f, 133, 220n2; "ever use" of, 4, 133, 208n10; extended-regime pills, 10–11, 14–15t, 17, 204; and family planning, 133–34, 135; interviewees' accounts of, 46; Microvlar, 14–15t, 120; new hormonal methods seen as unrelated to, 161; noncompliant use of, 18, 98, 133, 153, 220n2; norethisterone, 78, 208n9; Ortho-Novum, 8, 10f; rates of use, 207n5; repackaging of, 4; risks of, 208n10; Seasonale, 3, 4, 10, 181; uses of, 174; and weight loss, 132, 148, 180–81; Yasmin, 14–15t, 148, 180–81, 208n9, 219n23, 220n16

Organon-Brasil (pharmaceutical company), 160

Ortho Evra (hormonal patch), 4, 83

Ortho-Novum (oral contraceptive), 8, 10f

osteoporosis, 169

Oudshoorn, Nelly, 11–12, 106, 132, 161

ova donors, 125, 216n13

ovaries, 50, 88, 172

ovulation, 45, 50

pain, 89

PAISM (Women's Comprehensive Health Care Program), 32

Paleofantasy: What Evolution Really Tells Us about Sex, Diet and How We Live (Zuk), 101

Papua New Guinea: bodily substances in, 122, 215n15; bodily topology in, 63

Parés, Luis Nicolau, 22

Parker, Richard, 24–25

patients: and good/bad distinction, 137–39; patient–doctor relationships, 138–41, 158; rights of, 129, 138, 157

Pedro, Joana Maria, 134

Perpétuo, Ignez, 134

personalization of biomedical interventions, 130, 132, 136, 145, 148–49; and class, 150–54; and farmácias de manipulação, 163–65

Peterson, Kristin, 162

pharmaceutical anthropology, 175–80

pharmaceutical citizenship, 132–33

pharmaceutical corporations, 14t; data held by, 156; fieldwork at, 21; marketing of hormones by, 160, 180–81, 219n1, 219n23; marketing of implants by, 169; marketing of menstrual suppression by, 71; and packaging of hormones, 174–75, 220–21n16; and regulation of pharmacies, 164–65

pharmaceutical leakage, 19

pharmaceuticals/chemicals: absorption of, 40, 177; efficacy of, 180; as informed materials, 162–63; manufacture of, 163–68; marketing of, 180–81; materiality of, 177–80; packaging of, 174–75; similarity of to one another, 86, 159–61; symbolic efficacy of, 176–77; used in nonprescribed ways, 18, 98, 133, 153, 220n2. See also specific pharmaceuticals

Pharmacia-Upjohn, 134–35, 208n10

pharmacists: language used by, 115; manufacture of implants by, 165–67

phenomenology, 40, 52, 179

pheromones, 170

pill, the. See oral contraceptives

placebo pills, 8–10

Plan B (emergency contraceptive), 159

plasticity, 188, 189–90; in Bahia, 197; of the body, 6, 101–2, 190–92, 193, 197; cost of, 202–3; and flexibility, 40–41, 199–200; importance of, 201–2; meanings of, 40–41, 193, 199–201;

TPM (*tensão premenstrual*). *See* premenstrual tension (PMT)
transsexuals. *See travestis*
Travesti Association of Salvador (ATRAS), 21, 109–11, 123–24
travestis: access to health care by, 109, 111; availability of hormones to, 105; as distinct from transsexuals, 124, 215n1; and *hormônio* as substance, 123–24; knowledge about hormones, 116; use of *hormônio* by, 108–11; use of term, 21, 215n1
triage, 29, 133, 142–44
tubal ligations. *See* sterilization, female

United States: Depo-Provera approval in, 217n6; drug packaging in, 175; images of menstrual suppression in, 74–75; modes of biomedical living in, 28
USAID, 134–35, 136
uterus, the: in biomedical literature, 76–77; as disposable, 95, 120, 121; imaging of, 51, 77; sense perception of, 50–52; surgeries on, 77–78. *See also* hysterectomies

vaginas: and bodily boundaries, 63–65; and modernity, 29; and natural birth, 7; sex hormones absorbed through, 4, 160
van de Port, Mattijs, 22, 193–95, 204
vasectomies, 139, 141–44

Victora, Cesar, 28
Viva Sem Menstruar (Live without menstruating) advertising campaign, 71
Viveiros de Castro, Eduardo, 39, 196–97, 198

Walker, Anne, 80
Watkins, Elizabeth, 159
weight gain: as accumulation of menstrual blood, 120; as hormonally induced, 16, 115, 148; and implants, 96, 117. *See also* swelling
weight loss: and implants, 171, 173; and oral contraceptives, 132, 148, 180–81
Weismantel, Mary, 35–36
"What Was Life?" (Helmreich), 192
Whitehouse, Harold Beckwith, 71
Whyte, Susan, 176
Women's Comprehensive Health Care Program (PAISM), 32
Wong, Laura, 134
work: domestic, 60; and menstrual cycle, 81–84; and PMT, 82–83
World Health Organization (WHO), 1, 12, 141–42

Yasmin (oral contraceptive), 14–15t, 148, 180–81, 208n9, 219n23, 220n16

Žižek, Slavoj, 200
Zuk, Marlene, 101